Reimagining N
Through Pra
Autoethnography

Reimagining Narrative Therapy Through Practice Stories and Autoethnography takes a new pedagogical approach to teaching and learning in contemporary narrative therapy, based in autoethnography and storytelling.

The individual client stories aim to paint each therapeutic meeting in such detail that the reader will come to feel as though they actually know the two or more people in the room. This approach moves beyond the standard narrative practice of teaching by transcripts and steps into teaching narrative therapy through autoethnography. The intention of these 'teaching tales' is to offer the reader an opportunity to enter into the very 'heart and soul' of narrative therapy practice, much like reading a novel has you enter into the lives of the characters that inhabit it. This work has been used by the authors in MA and PhD level classrooms, workshops, week-long intensive courses, and conferences around the world, where it has received commendations from both newcomer and veteran narrative therapists.

The aim of this book is to introduce narrative therapy and the value of integrating autoethnographic methods to students and new clinicians. It can also serve as a useful tool for advanced teachers of narrative practices. In addition, it will appeal to established clinicians who are curious about narrative therapy (who may be looking to add it to their practice), as well as students and scholars of autoethnography and qualitative inquiry and methods.

Travis Heath is an associate professor at the University of Denver. His interests include looking at shifting from a multicultural approach to counseling to one of cultural democracy that invites people to heal in mediums that are culturally near. He has been fortunate to run workshops and speak in ten countries to date.

Tom Stone Carlson is a professor in the Couple and Family Therapy Program at Alliant International University-San Diego and is the co-editor of the *Journal of Contemporary Narrative Therapy*. He has over 20 years' experience teaching narrative therapy and is particularly interested in the development of experience-near pedagogies for new therapists.

David Epston and Michael White (1948–2008) were the originators of narrative therapy. Their co-authored publications include *Narrative Means to Therapeutic Ends* (1990) and *Experience, Contradiction, Narrative and Imagination* (1992). Since then, David has (co)authored 11 books, and offered trainings around the world and in Aotearoa New Zealand.

"This book on contemporary narrative therapy re-embraces its inventive origins. It is filled with generative stories that at once re-ignite the imagination of therapists who have been vulnerable to the dictates of manuals, toolkits, and mechanistic practices that can paradoxically diminish the possibilities of the therapeutic endeavor. Accessible practitioner stories of narrative therapy and autoethnographic reflections take the reader on a journey into unmapped territories that awaken the spirit of playfulness, adventure, curiosity, novelty and surprise; the very lifeblood of therapeutic change. These therapeutic touchstones found throughout the book promote a refreshing look at the practice and teaching of narrative therapy that can invigorate practitioners and educators whose creativity and inspiration has been weakened by the rigidities of professional conformity. The text culminates with an intimate, aesthetically elegant examination of a new pedagogy in the teaching of narrative therapy that connects you to a sense of therapeutic magic and possibility."

— Dr. Gerald Monk, Professor of Marriage and Family Therapy, San Diego State University USA

"Since the beginning of human history stories have been passed on from one generation to the next with messages about ethic, meaning, care and spirit from the past that can potentially create relief and meaning to the struggles of the present. Our stories represent the essence of our lives. The gift of this book is like the gift of those stories. Reimagining Narrative Therapy Through Practice Stories makes you wonder why we for so many years have been learning practice skills through exercises, analysis, and models – when indeed the stories in this book reveal the skills and spirits of narrative work. With the words of Nick Thompson, an Apache elder referred in the book: 'This is what we know about our stories. They go to work on your mind and make you think about your life'.

The Authors propose 'an alternative pedagogy for teaching narrative therapy. Rather than propose traditional inductive methods of teaching a priori theory followed by the subsequent skills and intervention,' they 'propose a deductive approach that intentionally avoids the use of theoretical jargon or reference to any particular set of practices in favor of painting a picture of narrative practice.'

You will love their stories. Reading this book is not like reading yet another textbook on therapy. It will not teach you but show you 'the spirits of narrative practice'.

With this book the joy of narrative practice shows itself on every page. The authors put it this way: Stories 'provide guidance in a manner that inspires your own imaginative capacities rather than the provision of manualized and regulated direction.'

The stories in this book made us laugh, cry, wonder and think about our own lives. We can think of no better way to engage with narrative practice."

— *Anette and Allan Holmgren, Psychologists and directors of DISPUK, Danish Institute for Training in Narrative Therapy*

"'Show' outpaces 'tell' by miles—the tortoise always wins.

This edited book gives the reader 'practice stories' that show how narrative therapy works, instead of telling us how to do the work of narrative therapy. It has the unmistakable cadence of the narrative storyteller, and thus becomes 'travel companions' in our own practice. These stories allow us to live in an adventure full of creativity and ingenuity."

— *Dr. Victoria Dickerson, Ph.D. co-author of* If Problems Talked: Narrative Therapy in Action

Writing Lives
Ethnographic Narratives

Series Editors: Arthur P. Bochner, Carolyn Ellis and Tony E. Adams
University of South Florida and Bradley University

Writing Lives: Ethnographic Narratives publishes narrative representations of qualitative research projects. The series editors seek manuscripts that blur the boundaries between humanities and social sciences. We encourage novel and evocative forms of expressing concrete lived experience, including autoethnographic, literary, poetic, artistic, visual, performative, critical, multi-voiced, conversational, and co-constructed representations. We are interested in ethnographic narratives that depict local stories; employ literary modes of scene setting, dialogue, character development, and unfolding action; and include the author's critical reflections on the research and writing process, such as research ethics, alternative modes of inquiry and representation, reflexivity, and evocative storytelling. Proposals and manuscripts should be directed to abochner@usf.edu, cellis@usf.edu or tadams@bradley.edu

A Story of a Marriage Through Dementia and Beyond
Love in a Whirlwind
Laurel Richardson

Therapy, Stand-Up, and the Gesture of Writing
Towards Creative-Relational Inquiry
Jonathan Wyatt

Talking White Trash
Mediated Representations and Lived Experiences of White Working-Class People
Tasha R. Dunn

For more information about this series, please visit: www.routledge.com/Writing-Lives-Ethnographic-Narratives/book-series/WLEN

REIMAGINING NARRATIVE THERAPY THROUGH PRACTICE STORIES AND AUTOETHNOGRAPHY

Edited by
Travis Heath, Tom Stone Carlson,
and David Epston

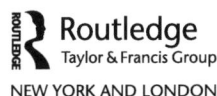

NEW YORK AND LONDON

Cover image: Getty images

First published 2022
by Routledge
605 Third Avenue, New York, NY 10158

and by Routledge
4 Park Square, Milton Park, Abingdon, Oxon, OX14 4RN

Routledge is an imprint of the Taylor & Francis Group, an informa business

© 2022 selection and editorial matter, Travis Heath, Tom Stone Carlson, and David Epston; individual chapters, the contributors

The right of Travis Heath, Tom Stone Carlson, and David Epston to be identified as the authors of the editorial material, and of the authors for their individual chapters, has been asserted in accordance with sections 77 and 78 of the Copyright, Designs and Patents Act 1988.

All rights reserved. No part of this book may be reprinted or reproduced or utilised in any form or by any electronic, mechanical, or other means, now known or hereafter invented, including photocopying and recording, or in any information storage or retrieval system, without permission in writing from the publishers.

Trademark notice: Product or corporate names may be trademarks or registered trademarks, and are used only for identification and explanation without intent to infringe.

Library of Congress Cataloging-in-Publication Data
A catalog record for this title has been requested

ISBN: 978-1-032-12864-1 (hbk)
ISBN: 978-1-032-12865-8 (pbk)
ISBN: 978-1-003-22654-3 (ebk)

DOI: 10.4324/9781003226543

Typeset in ITC Legacy Serif
by codeMantra

CONTENTS

List of Contributors   xi

SECTION I
INTRODUCTION TO PRACTICE STORIES   1

1   Introduction: Writing Practice Stories – A History of a Pedagogy   3
TRAVIS HEATH, DAVID EPSTON AND TOM CARLSON

SECTION II
STORIES IN ACTION   39

2   Wilbur the Worrier Becomes Wilbur the Warrior   41
KAY INGAMELLS

3   Mother Appreciation Parties   73
DAVID EPSTON

4   *"A New Surprise of Existing: The Last Thing I Ever Was – Was Silent"*: A Poetic Response to Patriarchal Malice   84
SANNI PALJAKKA AND FABIOLA

5   Blossoming in the Storm   117
SASHA MCALLUM PILKINGTON

6	Batman Returns: Love and Ethics in Narrative Couples Therapy TOM CARLSON	151
7	"Maybe We Are Okay": Contemporary Narrative Therapy in the Time of Trump TRAVIS HEATH	173

SECTION III
A TEACHING STORY 203

8	Inspirited Contemporary Narrative Therapy: A Two-Day Workshop TRAVIS HEATH	205
9	Conclusion: A Literary Means to Pedagogical Ends TOM CARLSON	262

Index 269

CONTRIBUTORS

Kay Ingamells M.S.W. (Auckland, New Zealand) has been working with individuals, children, young people and families since 1990. Kay began her career working with troubled young people and children in residential care and in specialist agencies, then spent nine years working in child and adolescent mental health. For the past ten years she has lectured in narrative therapy in higher education at undergraduate and post-graduate level and has been running a private therapy and counselling practice for children, families, young people and adults. Since 1992, Kay has been supervised by the co-inventor of narrative therapy, David Epston, and has taught alongside David since 2008. Kay has published several articles. She is currently writing and presenting about her apprenticeship with David Epston. Through a teaching collaboration with David Epston and Dr Tom Stone Carlson called The Apprenticeship in the Artistry of Narrative Practice, Kay provides one-on-one and group training to narrative practitioners who wish to develop their craft into artistry.

Sasha McAllum Pilkington works as counsellor for Harbour Hospice in Auckland, Aotearoa New Zealand. She has practiced as a narrative therapist for more than 30 years in a variety of contexts and has worked for Harbour Hospice since 2008. As part of Sasha's weekly practice, she meets with people who are living with a life-ending illness and their families, both in the community and in the hospice inpatient unit. She also meets with family members who are grieving after someone has died.

Sasha was first moved to write by the stories of the people she met with. She collaborated with them to create a variety of therapeutic documents including ethical wills, letters and legacy stories. Later, she began to write stories that illustrated narrative therapy to prepare practitioners to work in palliative care. She found in stories a powerful means of conveying not only questioning practices, but also the nuances of the unspoken.

The story in this book was written in collaboration with the woman in it as a legacy document for her son.

Sanni Paljakka is a Registered Psychologist in Alberta Canada and is the Director of the Calgary Narrative Collective (CNC). She is currently particularly passionate about her supervision work in her role as Director of Clinical Training at the CNC. Sanni is co-editor of the *Journal of Contemporary Narrative Therapy*. Sanni is the originator of a unique approach to narrative therapeutic documentation that uses poetry as a means to bring forth the counterstories of clients' lives. She has published widely on narrative therapy with a particular focus on feminist narrative ideas and practices. Sanni has presented her work in the United States and Canada and throughout the world.

Section I

INTRODUCTION TO PRACTICE STORIES

In this book, we propose an alternative pedagogy for teaching narrative therapy. Rather than propose traditional inductive methods of teaching a priori theory followed by the subsequent skills and intervention, we propose a deductive approach that intentionally avoids the use of theoretical jargon or reference to any particular set of practices in favor of painting a picture of narrative practice.

Practice stories represent a way of writing about practice that uses an "in the moment" storytelling approach to place the reader in the mind and heart of the therapist. It is a style of writing that is intended to be a form of artistic expression (Merleau-Ponty, 1964) that moves beyond a mere clinical description of practice in order to "awaken the experiences" (p. 19) of the reader and allows the practice to "take root in the consciousness of others" (p. 19). It is our belief that the immersive aspect of practice stories invites the reader into a relationship with the ideas and practices of the work, which creates a context for those ideas and practices to come to life for the therapist in ways that would not be possible through traditional clinical writing.

CHAPTER 1

INTRODUCTION
Writing Practice Stories – A History of a Pedagogy

Travis Heath, David Epston and Tom Carlson

Thinking with Stories
David Epston

Below you will find two stories. The first was published in 1997 in *Playful Approaches to Serious Problems: Narrative Therapy with Children and Their Families* (Freeman, Epston, & Lobovits, 1997) but in fact took place in the early 1960s. It tells of my father, who was known in the small Ontario town of Peterborough, where I (David) was raised, as "Benny the Peanut Man." Benny derived from Benjamin, and "the Peanut Man" derived from his occupation running a small lunch bar called The Nuttery, along with my mother, Helen, opposite the cinemas on the main street that also sold the peanuts he roasted daily. I wrote the second story several years ago but never got around to publishing it. It was a response to a problem previously unknown to me in my practice, and that was the vogue of young women binge drinking, their consequent over-intoxication, and the justifiable responses of their families when this was discovered, most often in ways similar to that told in this particular tale. By the time these families sought professional assistance, in every instance the situation was dire. I quickly intuited that this territory we all found ourselves in was unmapped.

DOI: 10.4324/9781003226543-2

Or so I thought. The following story has truly "stalked" me ever since I eventually figured out my father's intentions in my late 20s and my sobering realization that I had far from duped him. Quite the opposite—he had found a most intriguing way to teach me to know my limits. I was then given to consider how, in fact, I was the most temperate or at least the most prudent drinker of all my friends and was known as the one who could be relied on to keep everyone safe, much like the current designated driver. This was something I took pride in at the time and still do.

Story 1

"When I was 15, I informed my parents that I had engaged in underage drinking along with my somewhat older friends. My parents, as expected, took it pretty well but my father unexpectedly, did not leave it at that. Since he was a man who only drank on very rare occasions and kept little or no liquor on hand, I was surprised when he arrived home soon after my disclosure with a very large bag from the liquor store. On reflection, I suppose he chose an opportune time to start unpacking his bag. I observed him putting away bottles of rum, rye, scotch, vodka, and gin. In all my life, I had never seen so many different kinds of hard liquor in one place.

I couldn't help inquiring what was up. My father said he had been thinking about hard liquor ever since I had told him about my drinking, and he had got to wondering if hard liquor was as "hard" as it was when he was my age. I arrogantly replied, "So what's that got to do with all these bottles you've got here?" He said, "The only way to find out for sure is to try each kind out." I must admit to having been somewhat bemused. He invited me to join him in testing the hardness of hard liquor. "How do you do that?" I innocently asked. "Well, it's pretty easy, really. What you do is drink it. That's the only way to find out."

Now I knew I was on to a really good thing—free drinking at my father's expense. I had to laugh at my father's naiveté, considering the risks my friends were taking in diluting their father's liquor supplies with water to ensure their own supply. I had always considered my father a fool, so this was nothing new to me.

Every so often, my father would convene tests in which we would drink together, comparing the hardness of, say, rye whiskey when he was my age to its current proof. He would engage me in considering how "hard" whiskey was for me as we talked and drank together. We both got the odd headache, but that just went to prove how hard whiskey could be. My friends marveled at how I was duping my father and I seemed to gain a lot of respect from them for what I took to be my guile.

Many years later I realized that Benny's idea of "hardness" had a strong resemblance to the familiar concept of "knowing your limits." Benny had persisted with our experiments until he had gained sufficient evidence that I truly knew my limits. Because I had demonstrated my more carefully considered drinking habits to him, my father rested more easily at nights when he knew I was out with my friends" (Freeman, Epston, & Lobovits, 1997, pp. 185–186).

Story 2

There was a ruckus in the waiting room that quickly abated when I introduced myself to Roger, a man in his late 40s, Jocelyn, a woman of the same age, and their 18-year-old only child, Naomi. Roger looked apoplectic with rage; Naomi couldn't possibly have appeared more disgruntled than she did; and Jocelyn was pale with what I came to learn was apprehension. I invited them into my office. Before I knew it, Roger and Naomi had changed the seating arrangements from a congenial circle to something akin to a boxing match, each contestant in their respective corner, glaring at the other. I thought it wise to enquire what possibly could have brought such a situation about. It didn't take long for Jocelyn to have me appreciate their circumstances.

Naomi had recently turned 18, and Jocelyn told how "Our little family went out for a special dinner to celebrate" and how one of the highlights was their sharing a bottle of wine with Naomi who was now the legal age to drink alcohol. Three weeks later, Naomi had permission to stay overnight at her friend Tracy's. "Tracy is like our second daughter because she has spent so much time with us, even on holidays." That night the parents were roused at 1:30 am by a policewoman at their door and a policeman supporting their scantily clad, stuporous daughter who was reeking of vomit. She was so intoxicated that she could not stand up unaided. The policewoman sternly reported that they had found Naomi unconscious at a bus shelter in the central business district.

Jocelyn, who was a nurse, bathed Naomi, put her to bed and sat beside her all night to ensure her airways were clear of vomit. This event had seemingly overturned everything the parents and daughter had thought was so about the other. Roger and Jocelyn were alarmed at Naomi and "what could have happened to her" and said, "We just can't trust her anymore after that."

Naomi shrugged off her mistake but was incensed that her parents had grounded her for the foreseeable future. She quickly went on the attack by threatening all of the following: I am going to run away from home; I am going to leave school and get a job so I can support myself; and I am going to Social Welfare to see if I can get a youth benefit to live on my own because of our irreconcilable differences.

Roger and Jocelyn rose to this occasion and countered with threats of their own that had been informed by legal advice they had sought. This dispute had been going on now for two weeks and, according to Jocelyn, "It's getting worse, and I am afraid of what is going to become of our family." I had hardly said a word, and it was about 10 minutes into our meeting. But by now I had realized that I could not be an adjudicator, deciding on who was right and who was wrong without adding fuel to the fire of this rapidly escalating situation.

I held up my hand:

> Roger, Naomi, and Jocelyn, can I have your attention for just a moment as I have something I want to say to you, Naomi, and to you, Roger and Jocelyn? You will need to listen very carefully to what I am about to say. Why? I can see how this dispute has arisen from your mistake, Naomi, and your concerns for your daughter's well-being, Roger and Jocelyn. I do not dispute either your mistake, Naomi, or your concerns, Roger and Jocelyn. But tell me this—have you found over the past two weeks that no matter how either of you try to find a way out of it, you seem to be getting more into it? Naomi, I know you have tried your best to reassure your parents that the mistake you refer to will never happen again. Roger and Jocelyn, am I right in thinking that you are dead set on seeing that such a mistake never happens again? If I were to propose the means for you, Naomi, to prove to your parents that you know your limit, would you hear me out? Roger and Jocelyn, if Naomi were willing to risk learning her limits in your presence, would you give her a chance to do so? And would you be as rigorous as possible in seeing to it that she knows her limits and forbid her to go out with her friends until she does so?

Everyone was confused but at least I had their attention for the time being. How could I sustain it was now my concern. "Roger and Jocelyn, can I have your consent to speak to Naomi first?" Perhaps still skeptical, at least they conceded this opportunity to me. I knew I had to make the most of it.

DAVID: Naomi, what do you drink when you go out drinking?
NAOMI: Beer and tequila chasers sometimes!
D: Is that what you and your girlfriends generally drink at a bar?
N: Yeah.
D: Do you think you made that mistake a few weeks ago because you didn't know your limit?
N: Suppose so!
D: Can you even guess what your limit might be?
N: Not really!
D: How much does a beer and a tequila chaser cost?
N: About nine dollars.
D: Naomi, do you prefer imported or local beer?
N: What do you mean?
D: Well, if your parents were to arrange a drinking party for you and your girlfriends, that is if you wanted to invite them along, what would you want your parents to have on hand—Steinlager, Stella Artois, or Heineken?
N: What?
D: What would you think if I guaranteed you free beer and tequila for you and your girlfriends for going to the trouble of testing your limits?
N: What?

I knew this was high stakes, but that story that had resided in my mind for about 35 years. I had figured it out at age 27 when my father and mother had divulged this and other matters to me as well considered and planned. I will never know if they knew just how ingenious they were.

Not daring to glance at Roger and Jocelyn, I pressed on with my conversation with Naomi. "Naomi, do you have any jeans or anything with pockets that you would agree to wear at such a party?" "Why?" Now, Naomi was very curious by what seemed to be such a non sequitur. "To put the bottle caps in your pockets." "Why would I want to do that?"

> I'll tell you why. The day after, when your mum and dad show the home movie of you testing your limits, you can find out how many beers you had by counting your bottle caps. Because the only way I know to find your limit

7

is to go beyond it a time or two and then you can scale it back to your limit. Who knows what your limit might turn out to be? It might be one beer, or it might be 10. Only your mum and dad can tell, although you will also be able to decide by reviewing yourself on the movie of your drinking party.

Naomi had a wry grin, which I took to be part bemusement and part incredulity. But I was unconvinced she was taking me seriously.

Turning to Roger and Jocelyn for the first time, I asked,

Would you be willing to have a drinking party at your home either for just the three of you or, with Naomi's permission, also invite Tracy and her other girlfriends along? And would you foot the bill for the beer? Would you also arrange to make a home movie of the party so all of you can review it sometime the next day to see if you can work out what Naomi's limit might be? You know how a drunk often thinks they are much funnier and more interesting or capable to drive their car or motorbike, but when they to turn others who aren't drinking out of the same bottle, it is a very different story. Also, would you draw a straight line somewhere and ask Naomi to walk it for a kind of police test? I doubt if you could get a police breathalyzer?

By now, Naomi was looking more bemused, but Roger and Jocelyn seemed to grasp the gist of it as indicated by their very reasonable queries. I rushed to Naomi's aid.

Naomi, if you have any misgivings about this, just think of all the money you are going to save and if you make a mistake or two, your mum and dad will be on hand to make sure you do so safely, and they may know some remedies for hangovers.

Naomi remained uncertain, nodding her head from side to side, but at least agreed to go along with her parents in order to collectively determine her limit.

I now took up the matter of finding your limit with Jocelyn and Roger. "Would either of you say you know your limits?" They assured me they did. I turned to Naomi and asked if she thought her parents knew their limits. She told a story or two where Roger had exceeded his limit on special occasions such as family weddings and he conceded that this was so. "Roger, do you remember how when you were Naomi's age you learned your limit?"

INTRODUCTION

Roger became thoughtful, shaking his head from side to side.

You know, David, when I think back to my first drinking days, I am really ashamed of myself. Hey, I played senior rugby and, in those days, —probably it's still the same now—the after-match drinking was atrocious! You more or less drank until you dropped.

"How long was it before you learned your limit?" "Too long, David! Too long!" "Did any of your drinking mates pay a high price for not knowing their limits?" Roger looked down at his feet, ashamed.

I have never told you about this, Joce, but before we started dating, my rugby mates and I were at a "piss up." And Jim, whom I didn't know that well, but, hey, he was on the team, got the idea in his head to drive to Waiwera [50 kms north] to see his girlfriend. Well, he drove too fast around a corner, went over a steep bank, and died! We didn't drink much after his funeral. We had lost a mate, and that was the first funeral I ever went to. I always thought funerals were for old timers like your grandparents or your great-grandparents.

"Roger, is that how you learned your limit?"

Well, I don't know, but I never could drink the same way after that. Every time I thought of my mate, I would turn down an offer of a beer. So, I guess you're right. But what a way to learn your limit, David? The hard way!

Naomi and Jocelyn were respectfully silent, allowing Roger time to recover his equanimity.

Naomi, do you think a drinking party under your own roof with your selected guests, in which you can learn your limit and prove to your mum and dad that you know your limits, is better than running away from home, leaving school, or applying for a youth benefit from Social Welfare?

She agreed.

Jocelyn and Roger, for the price of a few cases of beer and a bottle or two of tequila, is it better to convince yourself that Naomi knows her limit under your roof so, should she make a mistake or three, that you are on hand to make sure she doesn't learn this lesson the hard way?

They agreed, and for the first time they all smiled at one another. After responding to a few more queries as to the details, they departed markedly less fractious than they had arrived.

The family returned about a month later. Naomi had insisted that the first drinking party be a family-only affair. "I thought my girlfriends might think it sounded too weird! But when I told Tracy about it after the first time, which wasn't too bad really, she asked if she could come to the next party at our house." She started laughing, looking at her father. "Actually, it was sort of fun with Dad! Tracy really loves my mum and dad. So, she was there for the second party. And David, I had her wear jeans, too, to collect her bottle caps!" She burst out laughing, followed by Jocelyn and Roger.

The parents related how Naomi had gone beyond her limit the first two times. But when I asked, they said they had expected this and didn't make a fuss about it. Instead, they showed her the home movie in which she had to admit she was losing her balance and "raving like a lunatic." They all agreed that they were almost sure Naomi now knew her limit, but they needed a few more drinking parties to be able to rest assured.

Jocelyn phoned a few months later to inform me of Naomi's limit. She and Roger had agreed to allow Naomi to go into the city with her friends; and although they did not sleep well until she returned home late that night, everyone was doing okay, considering.

Introduction

Why Do Stories Go With You?
David Epston

The question that has always perplexed me is how and why some stories stay with us and in a manner of speaking won't let us go. Like many of my professional generation, I was raised on Milton Erickson's stories that were collected by Sidney Rosen and published in *My Voice Will Go with You: The Teaching Tales of Milton H. Erickson* (1991). These tales reside with me to this day although I last read them in the mid-1990s. They were told and retold ad nauseum at workshops taught by Ericksonian acolytes and probably still are. I can only guess how many of those tales, which I had read and reread time and time again, engaged with my practice and found their way into my early publications (Epston, 1989), although I doubt if anyone who knew those stories well would have recognized that. How do they work then? I would suggest they provide guidance in a manner that inspires your own imaginative capacities rather than the provision of manualized and regulated direction.

I suspect that when these stories took up residence in my mind and played upon it, they began to amalgamate with the variant circumstances I and my clients found ourselves in and yielded very novel outcomes. But I have no doubt each one could be traced back, to one of those tales of Erickson's that had haunted me with charming ingenuity for so long. I thought with those tales and I suspect I still do.

Perhaps I could no longer recall each of Erickson's stories in detail, but I could remember the gist of each, or what I am going to refer to as its logic, no matter how counterintuitive many of the stories seemed at first reading. And that is something important about such practice stories: they do not reveal themselves entirely. Much is left as a puzzle that you cannot resist puzzling over. The best means I found to test the puzzle of a story was trying its logic out in similar circumstances. Practice stories show how to do things, but you have to figure out why. For me, what characterizes such stories is a lingering mystery that stalks me like a friendly ghost. I wonder if I were to indeed solve the story once and for all, it would no longer teach me. It would no longer be pedagogical. An exemplary tale must retain something akin to the magical lying somewhat beyond easy and obvious conclusions.

Writing Practice Stories
David Epston

I recently sent a PDF of a draft practice story to Jill Freedman, a friend and colleague in Chicago. Her reply was absolutely encouraging. "David, reading your story was like being there, sitting beside you, and seeing the family that the story was telling me about before my eyes." That is what the exemplary tale writer intends for their readers.

It should come as no surprise that narrative therapy might take a special interest in practice stories for pedagogical purposes. Surely, it would be odd if this were not the case. After all, as early as 1989, Michael White wondered in the subtitle of his seminal paper, *The Process of Questioning*, whether narrative therapy might be considered "a therapy of literary merit," a term he borrowed from Jerome Bruner (White, 1989).

I have used the term "practice stories" to describe this genre of exposition of practice since I edited "Story Corner" in the *Australian and New Zealand Journal of Family Therapy* over the period of Michael's editorship and a few years afterwards (1981–1990). With Jim Duvall's approval, between 2010 and 2018, I reinstated something similar in "The Corner" of the *Journal of Systemic Therapies*. Once again, this format encouraged submissions and publications in this exemplary tale genre (Epston, 2010). As well, it led to a series of special issues, first appearing as "Exemplary Tales: Virtual Apprenticeships" in *Journal of Systemic Therapies* (vol. 35, no. 2, 2016) and subsequently in following issues (vol. 35, nos. 3, 4), which grew out of the generosity of this journal to sponsor such reader-friendly and practice-friendly articles.

For so long now, practice stories have been well established and characteristic of the narrative therapy literature (Epston, 1989, 1998, 2008; Epston & White, 1992; Freeman, Epston, & Lobovits, 1997; Maisel, Epston, & Borden, 2004; Marsten, Epston, & Markham, 2016; White & Epston, 1990). In fact, practice stories have always been my preferred way to show my practice, whereas Michael's exemplary tale writing combined both showing and then telling by way of exegetical commentaries (in particular, White, 2007). We always thought of these as complementary genres.

Many years ago, I recall reading in the research literature what practitioners most often resort to when their practice is stuck. Formal academic research came last, followed by supervision and consultation with seniors, and then, perhaps counterintuitively, informal discussions with workmates and peers came first. It has always interested me that many of those discussions are carried on through the telling of versions of practice stories. Such a consultation usually is begun by a peer, who, after a moment or two of reflection, muses, "That reminds me of a person (family or case) I met with recently (or some time ago) ... let me tell you about it."

In agencies with long-serving staff, what might be called an exemplary tale-book becomes the joint property of the agency itself and is continually being circulated by way of such storytelling. These are stories that constantly get referenced, not with any expectation of providing explicit instructions or a manual on how to proceed but something rather different. Such stories circulate to show colleagues how their thinking might be re-invigorated once they appraise the parallels between the circumstances the story is telling about and the circumstances that have caused the therapist to consider thinking again or thinking afresh; that the circumstances they are now facing are beyond their experience—much like the situation I found myself in with regard to binge drinking and its consequences for young women and their families.

Some therapists might come to realize that the terrain they find themselves in is as yet unmapped and that they might have to find their own way. But perhaps others have traveled over similar terrain, had to find their way, and drafted a map while doing so. The two stories above, to pursue the metaphor of mapping and the unmapped, may overlap to some extent. Either one might travel according to the map implicit in their colleagues' or agency's story, travel along it until the specific circumstances force them to abandon it and find their own way, or decide they are on their own and for this very reason are intrigued by how their colleagues found their way rather than pointing to a way already in existence.

It is well known that oral cultures used stories as maps in which to repose knowledge of all kinds.

An oral culture's anthology of stories might be considered their archives or libraries. It is to such literature/storytelling traditions we might turn for guidance if we intend to do something similar. I have chosen in particular an ethnography by the anthropologist Keith Basso called *Wisdom Sits in Places: Landscape and Language Among the Western Apache* (1996). The Western Apache, in fact, refer to their stories as maps, and they sought Basso's help to write them down now so that many of them were engaging in the practices of literacy.

Nick Thompson, an Apache elder, describes how such stories work:

> This is what we know about our stories. They go to work on your mind and make you think about your life. Maybe you've not been acting right. So, someone goes hunting for you—maybe your grandmother, your grandfather...anyone can do it. So, someone stalks you and tells a story about what happened long ago. You are going to know they are aiming a story at you. All of a sudden it hits you! It is like an arrow they say. But when it goes in deep, it starts working on your mind right away. No one says anything to you, only that story is all, but now you know people are watching you and talking about you. So, you have to think about your life. Then you feel real weak, real weak, like you are sick. The story is working on you. You keep thinking about it. The story is changing you now, making you want to live right. So, you want to live better. It's hard to keep on living right. But you won't forget that story. It doesn't matter if you get old—that story will keep on stalking you same as the person who shot you with it in the first place.
>
> (Basso, p. 59)

What has intrigued me and some of my colleagues is how some practice stories have stalked us in a similar fashion, perhaps not so much to live right but to practice as professionals to the very best of our capacities. Such stories show us the way—the already mapped—or more aptly how to find our way when we reach the unmapped territories, rather than tell us as manuals or toolkits, to use two contemporary metaphors for training in our fields of practice.

This is why I write practice stories and have done so since submitting my very first one—*The Case of the Nightwatchman* (Epston, 1989)—to Michael White, who in 1981 was editor of the *Australian Family Therapy Journal* and who willingly accepted it for publication. In fact, that is how we first made each other's acquaintance. I was well aware that what I was proposing would be frowned upon by the style our professional ways of speaking and writing sanctioned and prescribed as scientific, neutral, or evidence-based. On principle, I objected to such restrictions, as did Michael, for the way that people were represented or under-represented or rendered sterile and character-less.

Cheryl Mattingly (2010) summarizes this style of representation:

Introduction

> The "medical chart" may be regarded as a narrative template for much professional writing. The distinction in literary theory between flat and round characters is helpful here.
>
> E.M Forster tells us that flat characters in their purest forms are constructed around a single idea or quality. Once identified as such, they never surprise us; they never waver. They are fixed. They do exactly what we expect them to do. They are in a manner of speaking "done for." Round characters, by contrast, possess multiple qualities, shadowy ambiguities, and outright contradictions. But most importantly they are capable of change.
>
> (Forster, 1927 as quote by Mattingly, 2010, p. 108)

Practice stories portray people according to their moral character as they engage with their plights by means of what matters most to them.

> Stories have the capacity to display and test people's character.... A story's characters are those who, in Bruner's words, exert efforts to come to terms whatever the trouble is. The story tells the success or failure of those efforts, or in a more philosophical talk, the difficulty in exerting success or failure. Stories have a singular capacity to delve into the character of characters who deal with trouble. Stories incite or guide reflection on 'who' these people are and the significance of being that kind of person. Many stories, if not most and possibly all, involve some test of character: a decisive moment at which a character's response declares what kind of person she is, or he is.
>
> (Frank, 2010, p. 29)

My intentions here are similar to those of Ruth Behar in her *Vulnerable Observer: Anthropology That Breaks Your Heart* (1997). Someday, I would like to trace the many variations on this in the practice stories I have published since 1981.

To write such practice stories, I had to find other styles, genres, and vocabularies by which such stories might be told. Max van Manen is a phenomenologist and qualitative researcher who has directed his theorizing to the practice of writing what he refers to as evocative, a style of writing and telling that allow for a text to "speak to us so that we may experience an emotional and ethical responsiveness, that we know ourselves addressed" (van Manen, 2014, pp. 240-241). He sums up such an enterprise in the following terms,

15

> There exists a relation between the writing structure of a text and the evoking effects that it may have on the reader ... The more vocative the text, the more strongly the meaning is embedded within it, hence, the more difficult to paraphrase or summarize the text and the felt understandings embedded within it.
>
> (p. 241)

He calls for a "poetizing form of writing" (p. 241).

Most accounts of what happens in therapy, when it comes to be represented in professional vocabularies and genres, sever what is presented from what happened between therapists and those who seek their help. These accounts are markedly one-sided. Such versions as we intend by practice stories require language that "authentically speaks the world rather than abstractly speaking of it as a language that reverberates the world," as Merleau-Ponty says "a language that sings the world" (Merleau-Ponty & Lefort, 1973, p. 242).

As Wittgenstein (1968) reminds us, "When I read a poem or narrative with feeling, something goes on in me which does not go on when I merely skim the lines for information" (p. 111). We experience the tone of a text not unlike the way we experience "the captivating effect of a compelling musical score or catchy tune" (van Manen, 2014, p. 267). As well, the aim is for the text to possess the empathic power to appeal, so that its meaning speaks to and makes a demand on the reader. Here we are looking for a language that is sensitive to the experiential, moral, emotional, and personal dimensions of professional practice and professional life. The attempt here is to try to reveal some knowledge in the action of the practitioner that are the sensual, atmospheric, and felt aspects of experience, knowledge that cannot be translated back into cognitive knowing.

This writing intends to "discover" what we know in how we act. According to van Manen, the reader/listener is stirred up, challenged primarily in the realm of the ethical, and provoked so that the deeper meaning of the text can have a transformative effect on the self of the reader. The reader might be motivated to think/feel very differently than they might have by other means if they should find themselves in situations that parallel those embedded in these stories which hopefully are not easily forgotten (see also Bochner & Ellis, 2016).

Introduction

From Manual to Story
Travis Heath

I was innocently whiling away the late afternoon in anticipation of the bell to announce the end of the school day in Mrs. Johnson's eighth grade advanced algebra class. My mind was preparing for basketball practice scheduled for 4:30 pm. Such reveries were interrupted by a stern voice referencing my recently submitted homework.

"This is not how we did it in class, Travis!" Mrs. Johnson declares in an uncommonly loud voice laced with what I took to be chastisement. My eyes look downward in deference. "How many times do we have to go over this?" she continues. "Why can't you just do it the way you've been taught?" I muster up the courage to whisper, "Because it's boring," suspecting there will be some measure of retribution for my impertinence.

If truth be told, I could do the algebra the way she had prescribed. After all, I had done it hundreds of times, but there had to be other ways to get there, right? Why did we have to take the same route every time? This habit of "freestyling" to find the same answer by different ways and means led to me failing my eighth-grade mathematics class. A big fat "F"! Such an abysmal grade was unprecedented for me. My parents were mystified. I was ashamed. This was my first really painful lesson in what happens if I didn't follow "the map."

This experience haunted me until the 12th grade, eroding any mathematical ingenuity I believed I had once possessed. It took an amazing teacher in my senior year to reintroduce me to math, which I had once befriended. After I demonstrated I could solve a problem the traditional way, she invited me to "play" with the numbers. Math became mysterious and fun once again. A college professor in my calculus class the next year furthered this momentum and actually reinforced what I thought I knew as a 13-year-old – there are many ways to traverse the terrain and find one's way to the "X" on the map.

Around the same time my math spirit was being shattered as an eighth grader, Epston and White (1992) were busy writing about the "spirit of adventure" in narrative therapy. I would not discover this work until I was a graduate student in clinical psychology a little over a decade later. "A spirit of adventure!" I repeated that to myself aloud moments after reading it. I rejoiced, knowing there was such a prospect. To me, this seemed like an essential ingredient in any healing practice. It made too much sense to ignore. Yet, most everyone in my formal training seemed to be doing just that. When I raised the idea of narrative practices to most of my professors or colleagues, I would get the metaphoric, pejorative pat on the head. "Well, that's not *real* therapy," they said. Or "That's more for social work than psychology." Despite their attempts at redirecting me, I remain undeterred in my conviction.

At the commencement of my doctoral studies in 2004, I felt like an explorer trapped inside a snow globe, seemingly without any way out. My mentors instructed me to retrace the same steps so often within such limited confines that the grounds before me revealed well-worn footprints that I was to faithfully follow. I was being asked to gently lead each of my "clients" by the hand along the same path without much consideration for whether or not the path would suit them in any particular way. Narrative therapy seemed like the only way out. I might have dropped out of the profession and left the field altogether if I had not been introduced to this practice.

Map as Manual or Anti-manual?

Some 15 years later, it appears not much has changed for many psychotherapies. For example, manualized approaches have proliferated. This is happening even despite continued evidence that manualized therapies are no more effective than non-manualized approaches (Johnsen & Friborg, 2015; Truijens, Zuhlke van-Hulzen, & Vanheule, 2018). These manuals certainly create the illusion of uniformity and pacify the requirements of quantitative researchers and insurance companies but have we stopped to consider what we might be losing by handing our therapeutic souls over to these kinds of prescriptive "treatments"? Do we risk losing the very humanity that we have long preached as being at the heart and soul of our practices?

For some years, narrative therapy has positioned itself as a kind of anti-manualized approach to therapy. Over the past decade, however, even narrative practices have fallen victim to the insidious creep of manualization. Michael White's *Maps of Narrative Practice* (2007) was an attempt to make narrative therapy widely accessible, which people from the outside often viewed as a form of magic that could not be adequately taught. It would seem *Maps* was his way of challenging the notion that the work was more about him as a person than it was about the practices. Michael's untimely death a year later positioned this as his last great, definitive work. Perhaps unwittingly, people in this neoliberal era came to view the contents of *Maps* as the way one is "supposed" to do narrative therapy, despite his warning to avoid such a temptation.

> I will emphasize here that the maps of this book are not *the* maps of narrative practice or a "true" or "correct" guide to narrative practice, whatever narrative practice is taken to be.
>
> (White, 2007, p. 5; original emphasis)

Michael instead proposed maps as something that "can be referred to for guidance on our journeys – in this case, on our journeys with the people who consult us about the predicaments and problems of their lives" (White, 2007, p. 5).

Did Michael's notion of "maps" become confounded by the "googlization" of maps in the same year and ever since? Over a decade later, might maps be masquerading as a manualized form of practicing narrative therapy? In their implementation of these maps, are teachers of narrative practice ignoring, even if unintentionally, the way in which maps are not neutral and value-free? Lacoste wrote:

> The map, perhaps the central referent of geography, is, and has been, fundamentally an instrument of power. A map is an abstraction from concrete reality which was designed and motivated by practical (and political and military) concerns; it is a way of representing space which facilitates its domination and control.
>
> (Lacoste, 1973, p. 1)

In reading Michael's work, it seems clear that he did not wish for maps in his book to be used in the way Lacoste described. He wrote, "As the author of these maps, it is important to for me to emphasize that I do not use them to police my conversations with the people who consult me" (White, 2007, p. 5). Would it be fair to say that Michael did not intend for his maps to police our narrative conversations as well?

Recently, a friend of mine invites me to a university clinic where he trains Masters students. He informs me, knowing my interest, that the program has a vigorous commitment to narrative therapy practice. Unsurprisingly, my excitement is palpable. I have often felt alone in the narrative community in my neck of the woods, and the thought of a formal graduate program committing itself to training students as narrative therapy practitioners has me positively giddy.

When I arrive at the clinic, I begin watching, from behind a one-way screen, a student working with a person who is beset with the problem of anxiety. I settle into my seat with an eager smile affixed to my face. I notice my friend remove a piece of notebook paper from the front pocket on the left side of his button-up shirt.

"What's that?" I enquire.

"These? They're the maps the student is to follow."

I feel my stomach sink. Perhaps I misheard him. "What do you mean?"

"You know, the maps of narrative practice?"

I try and give him the benefit of the doubt.

"Oh, is this something they created together in their last meeting?"

"No," my friend says with a little a dash of irritation.

"It's the narrative maps. You know, from Michael White."

I watch disconcertedly as the student faithfully reproduces the map of his teacher. I ask, "How did you come to understand that these maps would work for this particular person?"

My friend looks toward me, his brow furrowed with bewilderment.

"These maps work for everyone, right? Isn't this how *you* teach narrative therapy?"

I notice a tingling in my fingers and a fog overtaking my mind. How could this be? How could the very heart and soul of narrative practice have been extracted in the name of maps and training?

My friend begins to sense I am unnerved. "Is everything okay, Travis?"

I vigorously shake my head as if to try and break free from the spell cast over me. "Uh ... yeah. I'm fine." I don't have the nerve to tell him that a narrative therapy distilled down to a simple set of replicable techniques was a pale imitation of the narrative therapy practice with which I am familiar.

I flash a guileless smile, shake hands all around with staff and students, and wander out of the clinic into the crisp evening air. Although my office is just a short stroll away, I walk for an hour through the city trying to make sense of what I've just experienced. I fail to make any headway in my deliberations.

A couple of weeks later I reengage my friend. I explain some of my reservations of using maps to teach narrative therapy in this way. His reply is one that still travels with me to this day.

> Well, how can you teach something without scaffolding? We have to give students very clear directions of how to proceed and tangible things they can grab onto. It's great that you can do this creative thing that you do, but not everyone can do that, Trav. In fact, most people can't. We have to teach a kind of narrative therapy that everyone can practice, you know?

This moment changed the trajectory of my teaching, and I am grateful for my friend's comment. It became patently obvious that we needed an alternative way to teach narrative therapy, a way that honored the spirit of adventure that David and Michael cherished. While I didn't have an immediate answer, I knew there had to be a way to apprentice people in narrative practice that honored the spirit of dynamic co-creation. I was now on a mission to find it, or perhaps better said, help to create it.

Critical cartography speaks of mapping artists who engage in a process of counter-mapping (Wood, 2006). "Map artists do not reject maps. They reject the authority claimed by normative maps uniquely to portray reality as it is, that is, with dispassion and objectivity" (Wood, 2006, p. 10). Might it be possible that Michael was presenting *Maps of Narrative Practice* as the work of a mapping artist,[1] and the therapeutic community at large has translated it through the lens of traditional cartography and the more recent googlization that demands an obedience to the map? Has the effect of this actually dispirited the spirit of adventure proposed for narrative therapy? If this is so, what alternative pedagogies might recuperate an inspirited narrative therapy? This book represents our search for just such a pedagogy for teaching and learning narrative therapy.

Introduction

Autoethnography as Pedagogy for Teaching Inspirited Narrative Practices

> I shall be derelict. I leave methods to the botanists and mathematicians. There is a point at which methods devour themselves.
>
> (Fanon, 1967, p. 14)

Perhaps my friend in the previous story raised a valid question. How does one teach without first "installing" scaffolding for learners? Certainly, traditional pedagogies rely on this approach. What if the process could be reverse engineered? Could being swept away and enthralled by a story of therapeutic practice before opening a book on theory help foster a different kind of learning?

Understandings are embedded in practice and they come to life by seeing and feeling them first prior to "thinking" them in some form of order or rubric, and not by way of rules and regulations but what we refer to as "the spirits of practice." This goes along with Gilbert Ryle's classic distinction between "knowing that" and "knowing how" (1945). He suggests that one comes to knowledge from the grounds of practice up, not theory/professional standards of practice down. This is learning by way of apprenticeship, whereby the apprentice comes to acquire what Grasseni (2004) refers to as "skilled vision." Different ways of looking yield different ways of knowing. They see different worlds in front of their eyes because they were trained to see them. This is at variance to the "professional gaze" which has "become synonymous for an ethnocentric, hegemonic ways of exercising vision, imbued with rationalism" (p. 216). As an antidote, we have chosen the term "spirits of practice" to waylay anyone from grand schemes but instead encourage apprentices to pay close attention to actual practices which are revealed to the apprentice as their own embodied knowledge.

As Ingold (2000) explained, "Through repeated trials, and guided by his observations [the novice] gradually gets the 'feel' of things for himself—that is, he learns to fine-tune his own movements so as to achieve the rhythmic fluency of the accomplished practitioner" (p. 353). If this is so, might faithfully adhering to *the* map or the manual hinder a learner from developing a "feel for" rather than an "obedience to" narrative therapy practice?

While the prevalence of maps has seemingly increased as a rubric for training narrative therapists, especially in graduate programs, narrative therapy has a long history of teaching via videos, live interviews, and transcripts. While there is merit in these approaches from a technical perspective, they can miss the heart and soul of the process. For example, what is the therapist thinking or feeling from moment to moment in a therapeutic conversation? What are they apprehensive about? What is their internal dialogue? In what ways are they feeling closer to or more distant from their conversational partner? What are they thinking about in between conversations that might follow them into the therapy room? Transcripts and other examples of practice provide only the words spoken between the two people in conversation. These words are somewhat inert, like the text of a play before the lines are taken up and enacted and brought to life. How much of the therapeutic process is missed as a result of centering only the words that have been spoken? How much of the behind-the-scenes preparation that yields those words from the therapist is unavailable to learners in a transcript alone?

Introduction

Searching for a Story in Narrative Therapy

Early in my development as a narrative therapist I attended quite a number of conferences where this centering of the technical to the near exclusion of the heart and soul left me feeling as though narrative practices were only for people smarter than me.

As the erudite presenter goes through another line of transcript, I feel my eyes grow weary. He is talking with such conviction that I feel a little guilty for zoning out. It is as though he is performing some sort of intellectual or theoretical surgery on the words, and it is hard for me to translate any of this to my practice. His polysyllabic language starts to merge into a jumbled mess.

What is wrong with me? Are others around me just as bored? Maybe I'm not as smart as this sage on the stage, I think, but this presentation has no soul. Where is the humanity in this? Where are the people?

As I wander out of the room, pretending I have to use the restroom, I stare at the patterns of the wall outside the hotel ballroom. I dance a bored jig down the hallway. Finally, I arrive at the bathroom door, drop my right shoulder against it to push it open, and walk over to the mirror. I rub my eyes while staring at myself for a good five seconds. Maybe I'm just not cut out to be a therapist, doubt whispers in my ear. As a second-year PhD student I wonder how I hadn't figured this out sooner, and I'm left shaking my head and chuckling aloud at my own stupidity. Furthermore, I am baffled as well as miffed at spending another $300 at a conference which purported to assist me in becoming a better therapist. I take a small measure of solace in the fact that the university had paid the registration fee, but I still feel as though I'm fatally flawed wishing I, too, could smile and nod like the other attendees who are apparently cracking some kind of therapeutic code to which I'm just not privy.

I opt not to go back into the presentation. Fuck it, I think. I've seen this all before. I wander out into the streets of this foreign city where the conference is being held. I make a quick calculation in my head about how far I might need to walk to be far enough away that no one from the conference will 'out me' for playing hooky. I walk down the crowded streets weaving in and out of the mass of humanity until I find a coffee shop about a mile from the venue. I find a small table in the corner, sling my bag off my left shoulder, and breathe a sigh of relief. I reach into my bag and remove a book by a psychiatrist Irvin Yalom entitled *Staring at the*

Sun (2008). Having started to read it on the flight the day before, on the recommendation of a friend, I find myself intrigued enough after a brief introductory reading to reopen it. I pull out the receipt I was using as a hasty bookmark, thinking I might read for 5 or 10 minutes to focus my mind, something I have done since I was a child. The text has other plans. While reading, I find myself transported into the intimacy of a therapeutic conversation. When I worry as to the propriety of my presence in such an intimacy, I find myself welcome without any expectations other than to be attentive. Yalom has a way of taking people who are often, by virtue of the constraints of professionalized storytelling, described in only two dimensions and through his words opens up third, fourth, and fifth dimensions of possibility. I feel invested in the outcome. The therapeutic drama makes the book too tantalizing to put down.

Nearly 60 minutes later my trance is broken by a nearby voice asking, "What are you reading?" Taken aback, I fumble over my words trying to construct a reply, "What? Oh, this? Yeah, it's a book by Irv Yalom. It's about death anxiety and therapy and stuff." I figure he would have little interest in such a niche genre. "Nice! I love Yalom!" he declares. As he leans in just a little bit closer to look down at my book, I see a badge dangling from his neck. I glance at it without trying to be obvious. My stomach drops when I notice he is attending the very same conference. I feel flustered this is just kind of encounter I am seeking to avoid. "Hey, weren't you at the narrative therapy conference?" he inquires. My stomach sinks further. "Uh, yeah," I respond with an apprehension I am trying to mask. "Kind of makes you wonder why we spend all this money on conferences when we could just read Yalom's books," he quips with a large smile. "Hey, I've got to go back to meet someone at the hotel after I pick up a coffee. Maybe we can catch up later?" he asks. Trying to fake an enthusiasm I wasn't feeling as I customarily do in such awkward situations, I reply, "Okay, yeah, that would be cool." With that, he is gone.

Already feeling socially and emotionally exhausted, I spend the night reading in my hotel room. So, there is no catching up with the coffee shop confrère. However, his words stake claim to the lion's share of my mind. Why am I attending all of these conferences when reading Yalom's depictions of therapy via the written word seem to offer me so much more? Who decided that we should teach therapy with all technique and very little soul in much the same way I would imagine one might teach a mechanic to work on a car? How have we concluded that just the words

Introduction

of the therapist and the client in a transcript or hearing them on a grainy videotape are sufficient to help aspiring therapists understand all that is present in such an interaction? This moment in my hotel room in 2005 is my first glance through an autoethnographic window and the potential that stories can have in giving life to therapeutic conversations that transcripts and even videotapes cannot adequately portray.

Autoethnography and the Soul of Practice

It is likely that most narrative therapists aren't familiar with the method of autoethnography as it isn't taught in any formal narrative therapy training programs of which we are aware. Perhaps we might consider narrative therapy and autoethnography as like-minded and like-spirited. They are two approaches that have only come to know one another well after having found their respective ways – one to a practice of therapy and the other to a practice of qualitative research. Interestingly, when David read Art Bochner's book, *Coming to Narrative: A Personal History of Paradigm Change in the Human Sciences*, he realized their reading lists were virtually identical. The works of Mikhail Bakhtin, Gregory Bateson, Jerome Bruner, and Oliver Sacks had been read many times by both.

While there are a number of definitions of autoethnography, we have adopted the approach by Art Bochner and Carolyn Ellis that they have named "evocative autoethnography." It's a first-person approach that seeks to show rather than tell. It allows the researcher or, in our case, the therapist, to be written into the story. It doesn't treat the client as an object of study, but rather, as a co-author. As Bochner and Ellis (2016) wrote, "In retrospect, the change we wanted to make doesn't seem radical. We simply were acknowledging that researchers live in the world, too" (p. 50). What might be the implications in the teaching of psychotherapy to acknowledge that therapists also live in the world? How might it help people learn if the stories pulled back the curtain of the therapist's inner-world as therapeutic conversations unfolded?

Bochner and Ellis (2016) describe using story-telling as "a method for inviting readers to put themselves in our place" (p. 71). In this way, we hope the stories in this book can be used to apprentice, not just through theory or transcripts, but rather, by being taken inside the moment-to-moment emotional landscape of the therapist. Like Bochner and Ellis, we aspire to help readers engage with our stories morally, aesthetically, emotionally, and intellectually. If this endeavor is successful, perhaps the practice can begin to get under the skin of therapists learning narrative practice in ways they may not even be aware of until in conversation with a client of their own. As Mair (1988) writes, "We are in the story, and the story is in us... The story gives us eyes and ears attuned to the events that are shaped, not only by the story line, but by the whole atmosphere of its world" (pp. 128–129).

We've observed that the kinds of stories contained in this book are not accessed in a therapeutic conversation by a therapist in an intellectual way. That is, therapists don't *think* about what a therapist did in a technical sense in a given situation. Rather, the stories lead to a felt sense of a direction that might be worth traveling. As Ana Huerta-Lopez, a former student of this pedagogy said,

> These stories became companions to me in my work with my own clients. In fact, the stories and the people in them seemed to show up when I needed them most. The funny thing is that I didn't have to do anything to conjure them up. I carried them with me in my heart. As a result, I began to worry less and less about asking the right kind of narrative questions. I found myself guided more and more by the heart and spirit of narrative practice ... I had been freed from following a scripted or step by step method of how to do narrative therapy.
>
> (Carlson et al., 2017, p. 103)

It has not been uncommon for stories like those in this book to move readers to tears born of joy, moral outrage, solidarity, and tragedy. In fact, this has become one way for us to gauge whether or not the autoethnography truly meets the definition of evocative. Many of the authors of the stories in this book were surprised at how much people were moved by their stories in the early days of writing and performing them. I share this next account with some trepidation as it can risk sounding over the top.

In 2016, I was completing a workshop with my colleagues David Epston and marcela polanco. David presented the first day and marcela and I split time the second day. I share a two-part autoethnography about a young man named Ray (Heath & Arroyo, 2015, 2016). This is one of my first experiences with "performing" a story rather than simply reading it aloud. I am surprised by how physically and emotionally exhausted I feel while performing it. I stop every so often to query the audience: "Why might I have asked this question here? What work do you think this question might have been doing? What spirits of practice invited me to move in this direction?"

I'm lost in the performance and exchange with the audience and time runs away from me. I notice we have just 13 minutes until the workshop is scheduled to end. Unbeknown to me, I shift into academic, intellectual-mode. Not thinking much of it, I say, "I know we are running short on time. Is it okay if we stop here, and anyone who wants to read the rest of the story, please contact me and I'll send you a copy?"

As I look up and begin to scan the faces in the audience, I notice a good number of them have tears streaming down their faces. Others are removing tissues from their bags. I feel a rush of blood to my face. I fear I may have miscalculated the tone of my last question. An uncomfortable silence cloaks the auditorium. I have never experienced a workshop with this much ... feeling? I feel embarrassed that I didn't see this coming, and I'm not certain how to move forward.

A woman whom I have not met before raises her hand and asks with spirited conviction, "Aren't you going to finish the story? You can't just stop." A few other people voice their agreement. I reply, "I just want to be respectful of your time as I know it's been a long day." Another woman replies in no uncertain terms, "Finish the story!" Message received. "Okay, I will be happy to. Please know that if any of you have to leave at any point, I won't be offended."

I spend the next 45 minutes finishing the story. Near the end, I cry. I cry so hard that I have to stop reading for 60 seconds or so. I intentionally avoid apologizing as we, as professionals, especially men, are apt to do. Still, this is foreign territory for me and certainly not something I have done in front of an academic audience before.

I conclude the story. I take a deep breath and step down from the podium. The audience begins clapping as they always do in such situations. As I get ready to collect my bag and wait for the clapping to trail off, one person stands. Then another. Then a third. Soon, the whole audience is standing. This is flattering but uncomfortable. I'm not certain how to react. I flash an awkward smile and wait for the clapping to cease, all the while scanning for the nearest exit.

After I collect my computer and my notes, I notice a line of people forming, presumably waiting to engage in some kind of dialogue. I've learned over the years that a lot of these conversations are just an exchange of pleasantries or technical queries. On this day, the conversations moved in a very different direction. People approach me, one after the other, with tears in their eyes. They thank me for the humanity in the work. More than one tells me they have been reminded why they entered the field in the first place. They talk about aesthetics and beauty. I am overwhelmed. This is my first foray into the power of autoethnography and narrative therapy.

At the time, I wondered if this was just a one-off experience with this particular audience. Over the past five years I have continued to be surprised by the recurrence of similarly stirring emotional responses. I know that David and Tom have experienced similar response in their workshops using this pedagogy. These interactions have no doubt resuscitated this book on more than one occasion when we might have started drifting in another direction. The reaction to autoethnography as a way of teaching narrative therapy and its potential for apprenticing therapists interested in its practice became too strong to ignore.

The evocative and personal nature of the stories in this book offer a chance for the reader to begin a narrative apprenticeship with the author of each story, and in doing so, offer an alternative framework to the "classroom" where knowledge comes prepackaged by an expert who delivers it to students. Ingold (2001) wrote,

> ... if the knowledge of the expert is superior to that of the novice, it is not because she has acquired mental representations that have enabled her to construct a more elaborate picture of the world from the same corpus of data, but because her perceptual system is more attuned to 'picking up' critical features of the environment that the novice simply fails to notice.

By engaging with an adaptation of autoethnographic practice, in our storytelling, readers gain access to the perceptual system of the therapist which allows them to them to immerse themselves in the intimacies of the practices of each author.

Might narrative autoethnography allow learners to begin calibrating their therapeutic compasses even while not in the physical presence of an apprenticing therapist? Some early attempts in using this pedagogy seem to suggest this might be the case (Carlson et al., 2017; Vogel Mitchell, Heath, & Epston, 2017). One learner said using autoethnography to teach narrative practice "offered a nuanced glimpse into the art of therapy, and more broadly, the art of human experience ... this method of teaching through exemplary tales creates space to see theory applied" (Vogel Mitchell, Heath, & Epston, p. 83). Another added,

> ... a theory does not come alive in general terminology, but in the case of this (story) it looked crystal clear to me... I can most definitely see things in

(the story) coming up for me and guiding me through a difficult moment in clinical practice.

(pp. 84–85)

And still another learner concluded, "... I find myself more ecstatic about the potential of clinical practice than I ever imagined possible" (p. 86).

In terms of the overall value of using narrative autoethnographies

> students reported in their end-of-semester assessments of the course that one three-hour class using (this) approach was worth, in their estimation, 24 (a factor of eight times) to 48 (a factor of 16 times) hours of learning when compared to the traditional approaches

delivered by the same instructors (Carlson et al., 2017, pp. 96–97).

In the following chapters, there are six autoethnographic stories from six different narrative practitioners. It is our hope that each of these stories will invite you into the therapy room with the therapist and their conversational partner(s) and deep into the successes, challenges, and mysteries in their respective practices. As Bochner and Ellis (2016) described, "... readers become co-performers – you can think of them as additional characters in the story – examining themselves through the evocative power of the text" (p. 72). We hope this sort of intimacy will allow our practices to begin coursing through your veins and find you in your practice in ways that might prove to be uncanny and surprising. The goal is not for you to replicate the questions we're asking, but rather, for the spirits of narrative practice to join you in ways that agree with your soul.

For those of you interested in teaching narrative practices, we also include a chapter that takes you inside a workshop that uses one of the stories in the book, *Maybe We Are Okay: Psychotherapy in the Time of Trump*, to invite people into the spirits of narrative work. Epston and White (1992) cut to the heart of this idea nearly three decades ago:

> With regard to ideas and practices, we do not believe that we are in any one place at a particular point in time, rarely in particular places for very long. In making this observation, we are not suggesting that the developments in our work are sharply discontinuous - they are not. Nor are we suggesting that our values and our commitments are varying - they are not. And, we

> are definitely not arguing for forms of eclecticism which we eschew. However, we are drawing attention to the fact that one of the aspects associated with this work that is of central importance to us is the spirit of adventure.... What will be the direction of this evolution? It could be tempting to make pronouncements about this. But these would be too hard to live by. And besides, our sense is that most of the 'discoveries' that have played a significant part in the development of our practices... have been made after the fact (in response to...our work with families), with theoretical considerations assisting us to extend the limits of these practices. We acknowledge the fact that it is always so much easier to be 'wise' in hindsight than in foresight.
>
> (p. 9)

Rather than *talking about* how to teach approaches to contemporary narrative practice, in the spirit of the book, we will *show* a workshop in action. Again, the goal of this particular chapter is not to provide a script for teachers who might use these stories in their classrooms. Instead, it endeavors to demonstrate how these stories can lead to an inspirited narrative practice.

Lastly, perhaps some of you have picked up this book out of curiosity regarding the stories and have no formal expertise in psychotherapy or narrative practices. Please know that this book has been written for you, too. Our hope is that these stories will move you in ways that might prove to be of value in your life.

What Lies Ahead

So dear reader, here is a little preview of what is to come in this book. Of course, we don't want to give too much away but what would a good story be without a little bit of anticipation?

In Chapters 2-7, readers will find a variety of different stories of practice written by various authors and spanning several different topics and concerns that demonstrate their practice in action.

The first story (Chapter 2), "Wilbur the Worrier Becomes Wilbur the Warrior" by Kay Ingamells, gives an account of her work with a young boy who is in the grips of a life-threatening eating disorder. The story shows how Kay uses narrative ideas and practices to playfully engage his parents in an effort to tell a convincing counterstory of Wilbur's wonderfulnesses that nurtured Wilbur's mind and body against the hold that the eating disorder had on his life.

The second story (Chapter 3), "Mother Appreciation Parties" by David Epston, illustrates David's work with a teenage boy who had taken up screaming and insulting practices toward his mother that he had learned from his father. The story shows how narrative practices, particularly, Mother Appreciation Parties, helped this boy give an account of the effects of his actions in his mother's life and serve as a powerful expression of his acknowledgement of her efforts throughout his life.

The third story (Chapter 4), "A New Surprise of Existing: 'The Last Thing I Ever Was – Was Silent': A Poetic Response to Patriarchal Malice" by Sanni Paljakka and Fabiola, is a story about the reclamation of a life from the effects of persistent and ongoing stalking and public smear campaigns against a woman's life. The story shows Sanni's use of narrative practices such as counterstorying and the poetic therapeutic documents.

The fourth story (Chapter 5), "Blossoming in the Storm" by Sasha Pilkington and Chuan, tells the story of Sasha's work with a woman who is dying from cancer and how she navigates the heart wrenching prospect of leaving her husband and two children behind.

The fifth story (Chapter 6), "Batman Returns: Love and Ethics in Narrative Couple's Therapy" by Tom Carlson, tells the story of Tom's work with a couple on the verge of ending their relationship due to apathy and disregard. The story highlights Tom's unique practice of inviting partners to become intimate witnesses to one another's experience as a means for accountability in relationships.

The sixth story (Chapter 7), "'Maybe We Are Okay': Contemporary Narrative Therapy in the Time of Trump," by Travis Heath and Jane, provides an account of a dramatic encounter the day after the 2016 election between two people who on the surface appear quite different, politically and otherwise. The meeting starts with Jane's admission of voting for Trump and the story details their work together over this complicated political divide.

Chapter 8, "Inspirited Contemporary Narrative Therapy: A Two Day Workshop," by Travis Heath, attempts to describe this particular case story pedagogy for teaching narrative therapy. Consistent with the rest of the book, the workshop is told as a pedagogical story that gives an account of a two-day workshop that Travis gave using the practice story in Chapter 7.

Chapter 9, "A Review of Fortuitous Outcomes: A Literary Means to Pedagogical Ends," by Tom Carlson, is a non-traditional account of some of the outcomes of using this case story pedagogy in both graduate training programs and workshops around the world. Written in both theoretical and storied form, this chapter attempts to articulate the promise of a literary means as it relates to both intended and reported outcomes of our proposed case story pedagogy for teaching narrative practice.

Note

1 Compare Epston (2019) "He used 'maps' to reveal which way he is going and why he might head in this or that direction. At the same time, he warns there are so many directions he might have headed in. Or that you might head in. This is no manual ... no macdonaldization. This is an artist disclosing in the most congenial manner his mastery and his craft. At the same time he promises that one's craft precedes and makes possible the originality of the reader's eventual artistry" (p. 9).

References

Basso, K. (1996). *Wisdom sits in places: Landscape and language among the western Apache.* Albuquerque: University of New Mexico Press.

Behar, R. (1997). *Vulnerable observer: Anthropology that breaks your heart.* New York: Beacon Press.

Bochner, A., & Ellis, C. (2016). *Evocative autoethnography: Writing lives and telling stories*. New York: Routledge.

Carlson, T., Epston, E., Haire, A., Corturillo, E., Huerta Lopez, A., Vedvei, S., & Pilkington, S. (2017). Learning narrative therapy backwards: Exemplary tales as an alternative pedagogy for learning practice. *Journal of Systemic Therapies, 36*(1), 94–107.

Epston, D. (1989). *Collected papers*. Adelaide: Dulwich Centre Publications.

Epston, D. (1998). *Catching up with David Epston: A collection of narrative practice-based papers published between 1991 and 1996*. Adelaide: Dulwich Centre Publications.

Epston, D. (2008). *Down under and up over: Travels with narrative therapy*. Warrington: AFT Publishing.

Epston, D. (2010). The Corner: Innovations, ideas and leads. *Journal of Systemic Therapies, 29*(2), 88–93.

Epston, D., & White, M. (1992). *Experience, contradiction, narrative and imagination*. Adelaide: Dulwich Centre Publications.

Fanon, F. (1967). *Black skin, white masks*. (C. L. Markmann, Trans.). New York: Grove.

Frank, A.W. (2010). *Letting stories breathe: A socio-narratology*. Chicago, IL: University of Chicago Press.

Freeman, J., Epston, D., & Lobovits, D. (1997). *Playful approaches to serious problems: Narrative therapy with children and their families*. New York: Norton.

Grasseni, C. (2004). Skilled vision: An apprenticeship in breeding aesthetics. *Social Anthropology, 12*, 41–55.

Heath, T., & Arroyo, P. (2015). Spitting truth from my soul: A case story of rapping, probation, and narrative practices. Part I. *Journal of Systemic Therapies, 34*(3), 77–89.

Heath, T., & Arroyo, P. (2016). Spitting truth from my soul: A case story of rapping, probation and narrative practices. Part II. *Journal of Systemic Therapies, 34*(4), 80–90.

Ingold, T. (2000). From the transmission of representations to the education of attention. In H. Whitehouse (Ed.), *The debated mind: Evolutionary psychology versus ethnography* (pp. 113–153). Oxford: Berg.

Ingold, T. (2001). *The perception of the environment: Essays on livelihood, dwelling, and skill*. London: Routledge.

Johnsen, T. J., & Friborg, O. (2015). The effects of cognitive behavioral therapy as an anti-depressive treatment is falling: A meta-analysis. *Psychological Bulletin, 141*(4), 747–768.

Lacoste, Y. (1973). An illustration of geographical warfare. *Antipode, 5*, 1–13.

Mair, M. (1988). Psychology as storytelling. *Journal of Personal Construct Psychology, 2*, 125–137.

Maisel, R., Epston, D., & Borden, A. (2004). *Biting the hand that starves you: Inspiring resistance to anorexia/bulimia*. New York: Norton.

Marsten, D., Epston, D., & Markham, L. (2016). *Narrative therapy in wonderland: Connecting with children's imaginative know-how*. New York: Norton.

Mattingly, C. (2010). *The paradox of hope: Journeys through a clinical borderland*. Berkeley: University of California Press.

Merleau-Ponty, M. (1964). *Sense and non-sense* (H. L. Dreyfus and P. A. Dreyfus, Trans.). Chicago, IL: Northwestern University Press.

Merleau-Ponty, M., & Lefort, C. (1973). *The prose of the world*. Chicago, IL: Northwestern University Press.

Rosen, S. (1991). *My voice will go with you: The teaching tales of Milton H. Erickson*. New York: Norton.

Ryle, G. (1945). *Knowing how and knowing that: The presidential address*. Oxford: Oxford University Press.

Truijens, F., Zuhlke van-Hulzen, L., & Vanheule, S. (2018). To manualize, or not to manualize: Is that still the question? A systemic review of empirical evidence for manual superiority in psychological treatment. *Journal of Clinical Psychology*, 1–15.

van Manen, M. (2014). *Phenomenology of practice: Meaning-giving methods in phenomenological research and writing*. Walnut Creek, CA: Left Coast Press.

Vogel Mitchell, G., Heath, T., & Epston, D. (2017). A tale of an exemplary tale in-the classroom: An accidental inquiry of the restoration of beauty. *Journal of Systemic Therapies, 36*(1), 78–92.

White, M. (1989). The process of questioning: A therapy of literary merit? In M. White (Ed.). *Selected papers* (pp. 37–46). Adelaide: Dulwich Centre Publications.

White, M. (2007). *Maps of narrative practice*. New York: Norton.

White, M., & Epston, D. (1990). *Narrative means to therapeutic ends*. New York: Norton.

Wittgenstein, L. (1968). *Philosophical investigations: The English text of the third edition* (G.E.M. Anscombe, Trans.). London: Macmillan.

Wood, D. (2006). Map Art. *Cartographic Perspectives, 53*, 5–14.

Yalom, I. (2008). *Staring at the sun: Overcoming the terror of death*. San Francisco, CA: Jossey-Bass.

Section II

STORIES IN ACTION

CHAPTER 2

WILBUR THE WORRIER BECOMES WILBUR THE WARRIOR

KAY INGAMELLS

One Monday morning in the spring of 2010 I opened my inbox:

Hi Kay,
You were recommended to me by Dr Moiva who is a specialist in Wellington in eating disorders. My son Wilbur who is now eight has suffered from anorexia since the age of five. Could you please let me know whether you might be able to offer Wilbur some counselling? I would appreciate it if you would give me a call.

Thanks,
Liz

A boy with anorexia since the age of five? I had worked with many a young person carrying this most frightening of diagnoses, but an eight-year-old with a three-year history? Incredulous and in trepidation, I picked up the phone. Liz's voice began to crack as any loving parent's would as she told the tale of how ordinary childhood worries had slowly become more extreme and then assumed the voice of anorexia. Her mother's sorrow rose above and beyond her words as she described how Wilbur, desperate to shed weight from his already slender frame, had begun to run in circles around the dining room table after meals until he dropped to the floor in exhaustion. Despair attended her sorrow as she told me that Wilbur had also talked about taking his own life.

DOI: 10.4324/9781003226543-4

We made an appointment for the following week. Liz explained that her husband would also come even if it meant cancelling important meetings. I learned that Liz and her husband Doug were both senior research scientists. Devoted parents, they had first consulted with a psychiatrist. Consequently, Wilbur was assessed twice including an assessment in his school environment. The psychiatrist concluded that Will was progressing well and needed no further treatment, but Sue and Doug were unconvinced.

Session One

It was 11:03 am. My mobile rang:

> Hi Kay, this is Liz, Wilbur's mum. I'm really sorry, we're running late. Wilbur didn't want to come. He's saying there's nothing wrong with him and he doesn't want to meet you. We've been fighting to get him into the car. We're on our way now though.

I had already been approaching our meeting with some trepidation, wondering whether I might be able to help Wilbur and this family, so the news of his reluctance unnerved me more. I gathered myself as a professional athlete might do when, minutes before an important game, the team's best player has had to withdraw due to injury. The spring sun had blessed Auckland early this year and the day was unusually warm. I went downstairs from my upstairs office to the kitchen, took four glasses from the cupboard and set them ready on the counter. I heard the door click open. I crossed the waiting room, hand-outstretched, as is my way of greeting reluctant young people. I met Wilbur's eyes as he hesitated at the entrance.

> YOU MUST BE WILBUR, good to meet you. You must be hot after your journey! Would you mind helping me get some water for everyone?

I glanced fleetingly towards his parents to signal my welcome. On the strength of Wilbur's nod, I ushered him through to the kitchen, and placed two of the glasses I had already filled in Wilbur's hands.

> Wilbur, would you mind carrying these upstairs for your parents? You go up and I'll tell you which door to go through when we get there.

Wilbur unwittingly led us up the stairs to our session. I followed closely behind him keenly aware that any moment he might think better of it.

> Hey Wilbur, how about you put the glasses on that table over there, one on each side for your parents and then how about you sit here.

I leant down and picked up my basket bulging with richly colored pencils.

> Wilbur, have you ever seen pencils like this before? Have you ever seen colors so bright?

I made a few rough strokes on the butcher's paper I also had to hand. Wilbur stared at the bright strokes ripping across the page. He sank onto the cosy carpet in front of the table.

> Wilbur, you can draw as much as you want if you feel like it. How about you listen in as I talk to your parents and just let me know if there is anything you want to say.

Wilbur nodded, as if in a trance, pencil already in hand. Liz and Doug took their seats and looked expectantly towards me. Aware that unless I found some antidote to Wilbur's understandable reluctance, the meeting could be over before it had started, I gleaned my opening words from similar conversations with other young people who also had revolted against the idea that something might be wrong with them:

> Before we begin, I need to make sure that you haven't come to the wrong place.

Doug and Liz looked at one another, then back at me, somewhat bewildered.

> Let me explain... sometimes when young people are brought along to meet with me, they get the idea that there's something wrong with them and that I am here to help fix them. Very often this is not what parents think, but somehow young people get this idea. I don't expect you think there's anything wrong with Wilbur that needs fixing, although I appreciate that you are here because you are worried about him. I want to be sure that you know that I am not a kid fixer. I wouldn't want you to be talking to the wrong person.

Through the corners of my eyes, I could see that, while Wilbur's eyes were fixed on the paper, his ears were keenly tuned to my words. Liz and Doug looked baffled. This would certainly not be the opening they had expected. A knowing glance passed between them as they seemed to make the link I had hoped they would make to the phone call a few minutes earlier.

Liz exclaimed, "It sounds like we are in the right place then, because we certainly don't think Wilbur needs fixing."

Doug joined in, "As you said, we are all here together to help. These are not just Wilbur's worries; they are all our worries as a family."

Now that the way was clear, I proceeded.

> Liz and Doug, even though I know we are here to talk about what is worrying you all, will it be alright with you if we put that aside for a few minutes? I ask this because I find that worries often try to take over my conversations with people. As if it's not enough to worry people in their own homes, those same worries try to gate crash into this room and take over. If it's okay with you, I would like to know a little bit about Wilbur and his life when the worries are not around. I have a strong feeling that I may be able to discover some things about Wilbur that we can use together to pit against these worries.

Liz paused, then let out a bemused "sure." Doug looked at me, as if hoping I knew where I was going.

> Wilbur, is it alright with you if I ask your parents some questions about you for a few moments?

Wilbur's eyes immediately snapped away from his drawing and locked on mine. As he stared at me with an imperiousness more usual in a courtroom, I became very aware that this young man did not suffer fools gladly.

> If you want, you can just listen in, or you might just want to keep drawing.

Wilbur hesitated, and then gave me a solemn nod of consent before turning his attention back to the paper.

> Liz and Doug, can you please tell me what you think I will come to appreciate and respect about Wilbur if I come to know him as well as you do?

Liz replied eagerly.

> Well, Wilbur is great at thinking out ideas. He thinks of things I would never think of in a million years. Sometimes I just sit with my mouth open in amazement when I hear about some of the inventions he has come up with.

> Could you tell me a story about one of these inventions that Wilbur has thought up?

Liz quickly told me of Wilbur's plans to make a new form of remote controlled lightweight hovercraft which would rescue people at sea. I was about to ask more about Wilbur's intentions to rescue people with his hovercraft when an excited voice cut through my thoughts.

> I would send my hovercraft out when the waves were big so I could help the life-savers.

Quick to make the most of this opportunity, I changed tack.

> Wilbur, do you mind if I ask you a question about how you would get your hovercraft out to the people that needed saving? I know about as much about hovercrafts as I do about Rugby and that's not much at all.
> I know lots about Rugby.
> Do you? Do you play too or do you just like knowing about rugby?

Before he had a chance to answer, my eyes were alerted to a large number 12 on the back of his shirt - a rugby jersey!

> Hey Wilbur, is that a rugby jersey?

Wilbur proudly nodded.

> Can I ask you what team it's from?

Wilbur looked at me sidewise, perhaps finding it hard to believe that a sentient being would not recognize an Auckland Warriors rugby jersey.
"It's a Warriors' jersey!" he said indignantly.

> Hey, I'm sorry Wilbur, you must think I am stupid. Do you just like the Warriors, or do you like other teams too?

Wilbur relaxed as he began to take up his role as rugby educator.

I like the Titans, the Bronchos, the Cowboys, the Chiefs, the Crusaders and rhe Blues.

Hey, does that mean you don't like the All Blacks then?

A momentary look of scorn crossed Wilbur's face.

No, he said with scathing disdain, of course I like the All Blacks!

Your mum said earlier that you are good at remembering a lot of things. Would you mind telling me a little bit about what you know about rugby?

I know about Ben Matulino, and Simon Mannering.[1]

Really?

I know about lots of other sports too.

Like what?

Well, I know a lot about tennis and fencing because I play those, and I do hip-hop too at school, and swimming so I can be a life saver when I grow up. And I want to play cricket and basketball, and golf, and soccer.

Liz chipped in.

Wilbur loves sport and he wants to do all of them. He loves music too. He plays the guitar but wants to start the piano and the flute. We have to tell him that he just can't do them all at once and that he needs to hold back and try just a couple at a time. It's a bit like that with all his ideas. We have to try and slow him down or they can run away with him.

Hey Wilbur, " I interrupted, "do you think your mum might be right? Do your ideas try to run away with you a little bit sometimes?

Yeah, sometimes they take me the wrong way. They took me in the direction of the wrong team.

I must have looked a little puzzled because Doug took up the baton.

When Wilbur was playing Rugby last week he got confused and ran in the wrong direction. It was really distressing for him. It was distressing for all of us because that night after dinner Liz went into the bathroom and found clumps of hair clogging up the sink.

Liz joined in; her brow furrowed.

> We discovered he'd been pulling out his hair. Sometimes he does this when he's been being too hard on himself.

Doug gave Wilbur a worried sideways glance, as if checking to see whether he was able to withstand the conversation. Wilbur had seemingly retreated into the world of his drawing. I noticed the stiffness of his body and feared that I might need to steer the conversation elsewhere before long. Reassured by the tenderness of his parents, I decided to proceed a little further.

Doug spoke again now. His voice slowed as if he, too, was well aware that his words needed to be chosen with special care (he included Wilbur, even though his back was turned). Doug said that it had dawned on him that Wilbur's hair pulling could have had something to do with what had happened at the rugby game.

He said he had asked Wilbur if he was still upset by what had happened at rugby. Wilbur had replied that he thought it was his own fault and that he was dumb. Doug had assured Wilbur that he was certainly not dumb, that everyone runs in the wrong direction sometimes, and that he had done the same thing himself as a boy.

> Doug, do you think that maybe the thoughts took Wilbur the wrong way after the game too? Do you think they tricked him into going the wrong way twice?
>
> Yes, I think that's exactly what happened. It's like Liz said. Wilbur is really clever and has lots of clever ideas but sometimes it's like the ideas turn into worries and run away with him.

I looked down at Wilbur. I noticed that his body had slumped somewhat, and his hand idly moved across the paper without clear direction, making only straight lines compared to his previous extravagant forms.

> Wilbur, do you think the worry thoughts maybe took you the wrong way after the game too? Did the worry try and tell you that you are dumb when in fact you have lots of ideas and know about rugby and all about Simon Mannering and Ben Matulino?

Wilbur looked skeptical.

The Worrier Becomes the Warrior

I don't know everything about them, just almost everything.

"Okay," I relented, "am I right in thinking that you might know nearly everything, or if not nearly everything, then quite a lot?"

"Yeah," muttered Wilbur.

"Wilbur," I piped up in a lively voice, hoping I might lift the mood of the room which seemed to have slumped along with him, "Did you know that right there, at that table where you're sitting now, I talked to another boy once who told me that thoughts kept taking him in the wrong direction too? Can I tell you about him?"

Wilbur gave a nod which seemed a little more energetic than his previous nod of consent.

Do you have any idea what the thoughts did to him, Wilbur?

Wilbur shook his head.

The worries made him forget to take his underpants off when he went for his swimming test.

Wilbur stared at me in mild horror.

When I asked him what had happened, he said that the worry thoughts about the test chased away his concentration. Do you think that maybe his thoughts took him in the wrong direction at the swimming pool just like your thoughts took you in the wrong direction on the rugby field?

"Yeah, maybe," Wilbur said, then added, "Did everyone see his pants?"
"I don't know. But he said he was worried that everyone had seen his pants."

Do you think that maybe the worry tried to run away with him a little bit like those dumb thoughts tried to run away with you? Do you think it's possible that maybe, that's what happened to him too?

49

Wilbur's eyes narrowed. He seemed to me to be assessing whether I was leading him up the garden path and then thankfully appeared to decide to risk an answer:

> I guess.

Hoping to make the most of Wilbur's responsiveness, I asked another question.

> Can you please help me to understand what else these dumb thoughts tell you to do?

Wilbur was unequivocal.

> They tell me to be skinnier. They tell me I will get fat.
> Wilbur, is this another way the thoughts try and take you in the wrong direction? Do they try to tell you that you are fat when you are not, and try to get you to stop eating?

Wilbur was unable to answer. Instead, he began to crawl on his knees towards his mother. He climbed up into her lap and buried himself in his mother's chest.

> Wilbur, do you think you have had enough for today? Is it time to go home now?

Wilbur remained still; his face buried. Liz looked down at him tenderly.

> I think so Wilbur, don't you?

Liz looked across at Doug. A look of concern passed between them.
A few days later and email arrived from Liz:

> Dear Kay,
> Thanks so much for this morning. On the way home Wilbur asked, "How is she going to help me lose weight? Is she going to give me a pill or something"? Then he said, "She thinks that me being fat is a distraction for me." As if she is on the wrong path.
> I realize now we have a long way to go.
>
> Liz

Session Two (One Week Later)

This time, Doug brought Wilbur on his own. Wilbur, although a little less wary than the first time we met, did not return my smile. Instead, he settled down at the table again and lost himself in examining the colored pencils. I realized quickly that I would need to engage Wilbur through Doug.

> Wilbur, is it okay if I talk to your dad again, like I talked to your mum and dad last time?

Wilbur didn't answer. Wilbur had been on my mind since the previous week when we had met. Thoughts of clumps of hair in the sink and a bright spirit being misled by anxious thoughts entered my dreams. One night I woke with the idea of thoughts being like frightened sheep. It was this dreamy vision that gave me my direction. It also struck me, that Doug and Liz, like some other parents I had met, would be excellent co-therapists and without them I might not get far.

> Doug, I have been thinking about what you said last time about thoughts running away with Wilbur.

Doug looked at me a little bit askance but continued to entertain me.

> I found myself thinking about sheep. Do you know the expression 'Sheep Worrier'?

Before he could reply, I answered for him, concerned that I might lose the thread of the conversation. Through my therapist's peripheral vision, I saw that Wilbur's ears were pricked:

> A 'Sheep Worrier' is a dog that chases sheep. It can worry them so much they just start to run in all directions. They really don't have a clue where they are going and if they are not careful, they run right at the fences and get stuck trying to get through them. Doug, what do you think of the idea that the wild thoughts that chase Wilbur are a bit like the wild dogs that chase sheep around – or do you think that this is too crazy an idea?

51

Doug seemed to get my drift and took up the baton with the skill of a master therapist.

> Yes, I think maybe that's what happens. I know that when I worry a bit about stuff it's hard to hold onto my thoughts. It's a bit like I can't catch them and before I know it, they are running all over the place. Like sheep, just like you said. So, I guess this could be the same for Wilbur.
>
> Doug, do you think that when the thoughts are running scared like sheep that they can worry you sick and scare you silly?

Once again Doug ran with the idea.

> Yes, and it's like Wilbur said. If I can stop and concentrate, then I can calm myself down and usually I can find a thought to follow that's better.
>
> Doug, I just had an idea. Can I tell you?

By now, Wilbur was looking up, intent on our conversation and seemingly unaware that he was doing so.

> Do you know the best way to settle down sheep?

Doug took a guess.

> Do you mean by having a good sheepdog?
>
> How did you guess? That's exactly what I was thinking. I was wondering whether Wilbur could train these worry thoughts like a sheepdog would train sheep. I was wondering if he could calm them down and train them to go where he wants them to go, so they can't run away with him so easily.

Confident now that Wilbur would respond, I turned casually towards him.

> Hey, Wilbur, can I ask you a question? Will that be okay?

He nodded.

> Wilbur, do you think your imagination runs away with you sometimes and goes wild, just like when wild dogs run after sheep and make them wild with worry?

"Yeah," said Wilbur, "it goes all over the place."

Do the wild worries send you all over the place sometimes too, a bit like they did at the game the other week?

Yeah, I don't want them to do that.

Wilbur, do you like the idea of being in charge of all the thoughts so that they can't run away and become worry thoughts so easily?

Yeah, sometimes they make me late too, and I miss out on things I want to do.

Would you like to round up the wild worries like a trained sheepdog, stopping them from running all over the place like worried sheep? If you did that, maybe could you go in the right direction and get to do the things you want to do?

Wilbur's eyes sparkled at this prospect.

Wilbur, if you were a sheepdog and you had lots of sheep that ran away from you, all over the place, and they were getting sick with worry, how do you think you might round them up and calm them down?

Wilbur's imagination came to his aid as he burst out with a reply.

I would chase them really hard and bite them if there weren't listening. Then I would lead them to their cage and call the farmer. I would wrestle the sheep into that thing.

Do you mean a sheep pen?

Yeah, a sheep pen, I would like to wrestle them too, and nip them and bite them so they do what they are told!

That's good to hear! And if you got them to do what they were told, do you think you could have fun with them rather than being scared by them?

"Yeah!" Wilbur said with a hint of satisfaction.

I think I can see a problem, though, with you doing sheepdog training to tame these wild worries, Wilbur. Can you guess you what it is?

Is it that I'm not a sheepdog?

Yes, exactly! Do you think that you, me, and your dad could put our heads together and work out another way for you to train the wild worry thoughts?

53

Wilbur looked slightly disappointed.

"I know!" I exclaimed, in such a loud voice that Doug visibly twitched in his seat.

Wilbur and Doug, can you tell me what you have to do for rugby training? Do you need to train your body lots? What do you need to do?

Wilbur piped up before his Dad.

You have to be muscly, skinny and fast so you can get through the other players and push them away and tackle and not get tackled down to the ground so easily. You need really fast legs.

"Wilbur, do you have fast legs?"

Wilbur replied, with a puff of pride.

Yes, really fast.

Are you the first person in your family to play rugby, Wilbur?

No, of course not! Dad used to play rugby and my big sister played touch.

Doug, is this right? Did you play rugby and by any chance did you pass on your fast legs to Wilbur and his sister?

Doug again picked up the ball.

Sure do, or did, should I say. My playing days are over, but I played in the First 15s for New Zealand in my late teens, I tried out for the All Blacks before the Tri-nations. Wilbur's granddad on Liz's side and her father played for Wales way back. I was an okay fast runner, but I guess Wilbur's fast legs have come from Liz's side of the family. I was a halfback so passing and sidestepping were more important than speed.

Thrilled that we were on a roll, I kept moving.

Wilbur, did you know that your fast legs came from your mum's grandfather in Wales? (Wilbur had to admit that this was news to him). Do you need a strong body to have fast legs? Have you been working at getting your body strong so you can have fast legs for rugby?

Wilbur considered my rapid-fire questions.

> Yes, I need to be faster though and stronger.
> I don't know much about rugby so can you both help me here? I am thinking about how Wilbur can get strong enough to round up the wild worry thoughts and stop them running away with him. I'm not saying that he should try and train them all the time though, because they need a bit of freedom to run around. Maybe Wilbur might find that, when the worry-thoughts start to do what Wilbur tells them, they might decide to be imagination- thoughts instead and help Wilbur with his inventions. Doug, what do you think? If Wilbur trains his body, do you think that this might help him to train the wild worries that take over his mind?

Doug was quick to reply.

> I think my rugby training helped me to train my mind when I was about Wilbur's age, so I am sure it could help Wilbur to do the same thing.

Doug looked over at Wilbur. Wilbur looked back at Doug.
"What do you think Wilbur?" asked Doug.
Wilbur's nod shook his whole chest.
I jumped in.

> Great! Maybe we have a plan here. Doug, can you tell me what kind of rugby skills might be helpful for Wilbur to train himself in?
> Well, as I said, I was always a passer, so clearing from the scrum of course.

Wilbur piped up.

> Dad, you were like a sheepdog, weren't you?
> "A sheepdog?" I inquired. "Has your dad had training as a kind of rugby sheepdog too?"
> "Yeah," said Wilbur, "you had to get the ball and pass it, didn't you, Dad?"
> Doug chuckled, "Yeah, I guess I was a bit of a sheepdog."
> "Doug, are there any other rugby skills that might be helpful for Wilbur in his training to become faster and stronger?"
> "Fending," said Doug.

"Finding a gap too." Wilbur added. "And dodging and controlling the ball."

Okay. Now there is something else I don't know for sure, but I strongly suspect. Am I right in thinking Doug and Wilbur, that you need courage to play rugby? I mean, if you have a kid who looks like a tank coming towards you as fast as their legs can carry them, do you need to be brave? Doug, did you need to be brave when you played rugby?

Doug gazed ahead, seemingly reaching back into his memories.

I certainly did.
Wilbur, have you been training yourself in having courage at the same time as you've been training for fending and tackling and passing and finding a gap?

He admitted that he had had to be brave.

Wilbur, have I remembered rightly, did you tell me last time that your favorite rugby team was the Warriors?

Wilbur nodded emphatically.

Do you think that you could train yourself from being Wilbur the Worrier into Wilbur the Warrior?

As Wilbur's glance caught Doug's eyes, they laughed.

"What you think about that Wilbur?" Doug said through his smile. "Are you about to become Wilbur the Warrior?"

Session Three (Two Weeks Later)

The moment I set eyes on Wilbur, I had a strong suspicion that I was more in the presence of a warrior than a worrier. Somehow, he looked more robust. My suspicions were confirmed as I witnessed Wilbur pouncing up the stairs two at time to reach my room on the second floor.

Before the opportunity could slip away, I launched into the session. I directed a question at Doug, knowing that I might have only one opportunity and I needed to increase the odds of my question finding its aim.

> Doug, can you tell me if I am imagining things, or is there a little bit more warrior in Wilbur than there was the last time we met?

Doug caught my question in mid-air and ran with it.

> I think the warrior has been growing in the last week because of the training. Wilbur, can I tell Kay what I have seen?

Wilbur nodded.

> On the weekend we took this rugby ball, met up with some other boys and played touch rugby. I noticed that Wilbur was running between the two players. He used to run backwards or run away from people and now he can find a gap. I think that is a very useful and important warrior skill.
> Really!

Noticing that Wilbur's ears were pricked to his father's words, I decided that this was an opportunity to embroider this story of emerging warrior-dom. I began with a touch of intrigue.

> Wilbur, I have a hunch about what might be going on here. Is it alright if I share my hunch with you? I might be wrong so will you put me right if I have gone wrong?

Wilbur looked at me expectantly but with a hint of skepticism.

> Wilbur, has the warrior started to take control of your legs and send you in the right direction?
> Yeah!

This was a moment to be seized. I had found a gap between the two players in our conversation: the problem story and the embryonic counterstory.

> Wilbur, if your warrior has been starting to control your legs so that you are now going in the right direction, do you think that it has been starting to take control of the wild worries too? Has the warrior been rounding up the wild worries so they go in the right direction, not the wrong direction?
>
> Yep. And the warrior helped me at Adrenalin Forest too.[2]
>
> Really? Are you saying that the warrior doesn't only hang out with you on the rugby field? Are you saying that your warrior is brave enough to go to Adrenalin Forest?
>
> Yep. I even went on the Fear Fall and I wasn't even scared!
>
> Why is it called the 'Fear Fall'?

Wilbur replied with some authority.

> Because you fall down and it's kind of freaky. Well, for some people it might be freaky, but I was only scared for the first bit and then the freaky feelings went away.
>
> The freaky feelings went away! How did you get them to go away?

Wilbur informed me that he had been on the Fear Fall before and realized what the feeling was like.

> Ahhhhh. Right! Hold on, do you mind if I write this down. It seems very important to me. Wilbur willingly consented. Okay I am writing this down: "been on the Fear Fall before so knew what it was like.

I explained more as I stabbed the pencil onto my page for effect.

> Wilbur, are you onto something here? Do you think you may have discovered something about the freaky feelings that you might not have known before? Have you discovered that their bark is worse than their bite?

Wilbur nodded.

> Wilbur, do you think about this discovery you have made that the freaky feelings are dressed up worries? Do you think it might be like a warrior's

knowledge? Are you becoming wise like a warrior as well as strong like a warrior?

He nodded intently.

Yeah!
 Doug, what do you think? Is Wilbur becoming warrior-wise as well as warrior-strong?
 Yes, I think he is. In fact, this morning I saw a little battle between the worrier and the warrior.
 Really?
 Yes, I saw it before Wilbur went to tennis today.
 A battle?
 Yes, there was a battle going on. That's what it looked like to me. And the warrior won against the worrier this morning.
 The warrior won! Hey Wilbur, high five!

I held up my hand to Wilbur. Wilbur raised his foot instead of his hand.

"Okay, high foot instead," I said.

We all laughed.

Really, Wilbur! Did your warrior win against the worrier?

Wilbur replied, exaggerating his words.

Yes, the Waaaarrior won against the Wooooorier.
 "Wilbur," I ventured, "do you think your waaaarrior and the wooooorier have changed places?"

Wilbur considered my question, looked at me a little wearily and uttered a "maybe."

It struck me that perhaps Wilbur needed to rest. With my encouragement he curled up in the chair much as he had done in the previous session.

Doug, can I ask you a little about what you said earlier about being scared of heights?

Doug was a little surprised by my change in direction.

> Sure.
>
> Doug, how scared of heights would you say you are? An enormous amount, a middle amount or a small amount?
>
> Oh, a huge amount.

A voice piped up from the curled up cat-like Wilbur on the easy chair.

> Dad, you are even too scared to go on the climbing wall.
>
> Is that right, Doug?

Doug admitted that this was so.

It turned out that Doug had always had a fear of heights.

Earlier in our conversation I had tucked away an idea. If Wilbur took to it, I was confident this idea would help propel his warrior training forwards.

> Doug, do you think you might be in need of a bit of warrior training too?

Wilbur looked up and scrutinized his father.

Doug agreed with slight embarrassment that indeed he did.

> Would you agree, Doug, that Wilbur may be a little ahead of you with his warrior training, at least as far as the freaky feelings about height go?
>
> Yeah, I could help you, Dad.
>
> "Would you, Wilbur?" Doug kindly asked.
>
> I'm a bit scared, and I think I could do with some help.

A moment later, Wilbur had conscripted Doug into "warrior training" at the local climbing wall that very weekend, the weekend of Doug's birthday.

Email from Liz after Session Three

Hi Kay,

You have been fantastic for Wilbur and the family. Part of me does not think Wilbur is out of the woods yet. One week ago, I accidentally left my scales out because we are having a room painted. He got on the scales before going to school. From then on it was mayhem! He was out the front of the house, screaming at the top of his voice as we walked down the road "I am so fat! I am going to tell everyone at school I am so fat!" I told him it was his worrier trying to tell him he was fat. I did not show him how distressed his behavior was making me. He was a lot calmer when I picked him up from school and appeared to have had a good day (even though I had a terrible day thinking about it). So yes, Wilbur has improved a lot, but I hold my breath, thinking when all of this is going to resurface.

Liz

Session Four (One Week Later)

Just as Liz had not "shown her distress" to Wilbur, I too had withheld the quickening of my own worry at the reappearance of the specter of anorexia. Fear could have taken me in the direction of doubting the ground we had gained. Instead, I gambled on my hunch that as long as Wilbur's courage continued to outpace fear, despite its recent reappearance, anorexia's hold over him would continue to slip.

I asked my first question almost before they had touched down on their respective seats. My line of inquiry was contrary to what they might have expected:

> Wilbur, were you somehow able to pass some of your courage onto your dad so that he could dodge the freaky feelings, or did they get the better of him? I hope you didn't have to take him home again on his birthday?

Wilbur smirked and then a gravity took hold of him as he declared:

> Dad did it! He did it! I know he was scared because I could see his legs wobbling, but you did it, didn't you, Dad?

I looked at Doug. His face had tightened at the recollection of the ordeal, although at the same time, I could see his pleasure at his son's exclamation. This indeed had been a testing birthday event and, even if born of a concern to accompany his son through his own ordeal, this was no fake performance. Father had joined son in rendering himself courageous.

> Doug, since climbing the wall with Wilbur's help on your birthday, have you discovered anything about fear that you either didn't already know or that you had forgotten? For instance, did you find that the fear's bark was worse than its bite, or that once you had made the decision to climb, the fear had less of a grip on you?

Doug paused reflectively before replying.

> Yes, there have been times in my life when I have been so scared of heights that I've missed out on things that I would have loved to have done, such as going on some of the great New Zealand mountain walks with friends. At

other times I have defied the fear and, although still scary, it hasn't always been as bad as I'd imagined. So yes, its bark has often turned out to be worse than its bite. I guess it's true that worries can be pretty powerful and can convince you they're real when they are not always as real as they seem. I knew in my head that there was nothing to be scared of climbing the wall, but it took doing it to really believe this.

Doug, do you think it's likely that, if you hadn't tested the climbing worry, it could have become freakier and freakier?

Doug, noticing Wilbur's intensity, adeptly passed my question to him.

Wilbur, what do you think?

Wilbur pulled a face before delivering a home truth.

You know, Dad, I think you should have done it sooner. The worries started freaking you out.

Wilbur, do you think the worries turned your dad into a worrier and then, in the nick of time, he turned himself into a warrior, like you did?

Yeah, (once again exaggerating his words), he was a Woooorier and now he's a Waaaarrioor.

Doug, in any way would you say that Wilbur's taking himself away from a worrier direction and towards a warrior direction has helped you to do the same? Or am I making too much of this?

Doug was quick to reassure us both that Wilbur had indeed inspired him.

Wilbur, do you have any advice for your dad if any other worries start turning into freaky feelings and try to turn him back into a worrier?

Wilbur was ready with his sage counsel.

Yep, Dad, you just need to tell yourself that worries are liars and that you can be a warrior.

Confident that Doug was with me every step of the way, I asked Wilbur:

63

Would you be willing to coach your dad, like your rugby coach coaches you, if you noticed that there were any freaky feelings worrying him?

Wilbur nodded so hard he looked as if his head would fall off.

Doug, would you be willing to let Wilbur coach you?

Doug agreed to this arrangement and, to ritualize it, I asked them to shake hands. They did.

We had all agreed that we would wait to see how Wilbur's warrior-dom was getting on before scheduling another session. A month later I emailed to check in. Liz emailed back:

> Wilbur is in such an amazing space at the moment, we are not sure if he needs to see you again in the near future. The warrior has been winning and there have been lots of positive things in the last month. His doctor is happy because he is gaining weight and eating well. He's not talking about being fat and needing to be thin anymore. He's a much happier child all round. We are so delighted.

I heard nothing more for 18 months, so assumed all was well, until an email appeared from Liz:

> Hi Kay,
> I am emailing you with the possibility that we bring Wilbur to see you again. Thanks to your therapy last year, he has been going extremely well. He has grown into a confident and happy child. He has done very well with his schoolwork, his guitar, his sport, and his social life. The anorexia has not been intrusive, but there have always been some underlying elements there intermittently.
> We had a burglary earlier this year and, since then, Wilbur has not been quite himself and he is very anxious. He does not seem as content as he usually is, and even though he is doing really well at rugby, after the last two matches he has been sobbing, saying that he didn't do well enough and is 'not good enough for the team'. He is asking to see you again.
>
> Liz

Sobered by the return of the anxiety and the perfectionism, I pondered how to go about the return meeting with Wilbur. Although heartened that he was asking to meet with me, I thought it wise to continue where we had left off even although a long time had passed since we last met. I emailed Liz to ask for her thoughts.

> I've been considering a more indirect approach, given that Wilbur seems to shy away from anything too closely directed at him. I've been wondering about a further 'bravery project' of some kind which Wilbur could undertake with Doug. I thought it could center on researching family/ancestral stories of bravery. What do you think?

Liz replied.

> I think the bravery project is a good idea. The ancestral stories coincide with his tasks at school, so that is fantastic. One of my distant relatives/ancestors was 'Spot' Turner, a well-known gangster in the East End of London, and an accomplice of the Kray twins. Wilbur loves this story.

Session Five (18 Months after Session Four)

There, in the waiting room, was the same Wilbur I remembered, plus another ten or so centimeters in height. At the risk of Doug concluding that I had gone off the rails since we last met, I decided to begin audaciously. While I needed to mention the burglary, I hoped that bravery rather than the effects of the burglary would become the centerpiece of a conversation which would lead us towards ancestral bravery.

> Wilbur, it's good to see you! Your mum told me that you had the idea to come back and see me. Is that right?

Wilbur nodded, looking slightly uneasy. He responded awkwardly, looking down at the carpet.

> Yeah, it's because of the burglary.

Doug came to his son's rescue.

> Nowadays Wilbur can say when he is worried which is a big difference that we're very pleased about. That's how Wilbur came to ask us if he could come back.
>
> Wilbur, did you ask to see me because you realised that the worries could use the burglary as a way of trying to steal your courage back from you?

Wilbur took up my suggestion more readily than I could have hoped for.

> Yeah, I thought you might help me to get the worries again.
>
> Wilbur, when you say, 'get the worries' do you mean that you've learnt that the worries can be gotten, that you got them last time, so you can get them again, or do you mean something else?

Doug chipped in.

> We were talking in the car on the way over about the other week. We had been in the park and Wilbur noticed this baby bird which had puffed its feathers up so much that it looked ridiculous. We laughed because it looked so silly. Wilbur said the puffed up bird was a bit like the freaky

feelings – the worries had puffed themselves up to look very big and freaky but really they were not that big or freaky at all underneath.

Wilbur, is that right? Is your dad saying that the freaky feelings used to fool you into thinking that they were bigger and more powerful than they really were and now you can see through them?

Wilbur nodded, and then replied:

I did get scared about the burglary but I'm not as scared as I was ages ago.

Wilbur, do you think that your warrior training has helped you become a little bit immune to the freaky feelings? Even though the burglary was scary, did some of the Warrior-You stay with you and refuse to be scared off?

Wilbur gave me another "Yeah."

Doug, I have been wondering a few things about this bravery. Wilbur, do you remember when your dad was brave enough to go up the climbing wall on his birthday?

Doug grinned sheepishly at the memory.

Doug, do you think that Wilbur's bravery kind of rubbed off on you?

"Yes," he confirmed.

If Wilbur's bravery rubbed off on you, do you think it might also be possible that bravery can rub off from one family member to another across generations?

Doug agreed that this was indeed possible.

Wilbur, I've been wondering whether your bravery might not just be your bravery?

Wilbur looked at me quizzically.

Can I explain what I mean and why I've been thinking about this?

Wilbur nodded; his interest aroused.

> Well, it goes back to when your mum emailed me a few weeks ago. She told me about your ancestor 'Spot' Turner. She didn't tell me much, but it sounds like quite a story, and I hoped you might tell me more.

My intention was to see whether we might slowly graft the story of Spot's courage to Wilbur's own story. This was not a fool-proof endeavor, so I had other possible lines of inquiry up my sleeve.

Doug and Wilbur gave a potted version of Spot's exploits and how he had defied the law for more than a decade with his Houdini-like narrow escapes and had become something of a popular hero. Despite the nastiness of some of his exploits, he was also known for being on the side of the underdog. In a bid to begin to play with the idea that the presence of bravery does not mean that there is an absence of fear, but rather, bravery is wrought out of fear, I asked Wilbur what he thought Spot might have been frightened of.

Wilbur said he thought Spot would be frightened other gangsters might "revenge" him. When I asked whether Spot's bravery had cropped up in any other family member, the conversation took an unexpected turn.

Bouncing with excitement, Wilbur spoke.

> Dad, what about the budgie smuggler?
> "Budgie smuggler!" I exclaimed, in amusement (in New Zealand and Australia, a budgie smuggler is a jocular term for men's brief swimming trunks or Speedos).

Doug began to tell me how, in the 1980s, his second cousin, Paul, had flown a light aircraft smuggling rare birds from Australia to a farm maybe owned by an accomplice in the South Island of New Zealand.

At the time, New Zealand was being used as a transfer station for the sale of exotic Australian birds to other countries. This particular bird-smuggling mission was only the second Paul had attempted but proved to be his last. As family history has it, his journey across the Tasman, which ordinarily would have been risky in a light aircraft, was especially perilous on this particular night. The plane's engine was damaged after running into a cyclone just off the New Zealand coast and Paul had to make an emergency landing into the hay bales lining the makeshift runway. Paul leapt from his damaged plane, the birds chirping loudly, to find that he was met, not by his bird-selling accomplice, but by the police who had been investigating "Operation Speedo" for months.

Wilbur was rapt with excitement as Doug relayed the story.

While I didn't necessarily want to include criminal activity, even of the budgie-smuggling variety, into our therapy conversation, I wondered whether we might sidestep the criminality to help Wilbur tap into the vein of family courage. Mindful that being too direct might not work with the bright-as-a-button, not-suffering-fools-gladly Wilbur, and having succeeded in the past with young people by helping them to find their own abilities through connecting them to those of meaningful others, I suspected that the budgie smuggler might come to our aid.

> "Wilbur," I tentatively asked, "do you think Paul would have been a bit scared that night as he flew on his own across the Tasman?"

Wilbur's legendary imagination had been captured by his father's account.

> Yeah, he could have been chased by other planes and he could even have fallen asleep because he was flying at night.

Doug picked up where I had left off before.

> I am sure he must have been scared.

Noticing an entry point to extend the idea of courage as a practice rather than as an internal quality, I asked Doug what he thought would have happened if Paul had gotten away with it. Doug thought that Paul would most likely have gone on to other dodgy deals.

> If he had gone on, do you think that he would have been as scared as he had been in the beginning?

Doug took the question in the direction that I had hoped.

> I don't think he would have been as scared the next time; he would have known the route better?
>
> Wilbur, what do you think? Do you think that he might have been a bit less scared the next time?

Wilbur agreed, adding that he would have thought the mission through more, and although he might still have gotten caught, and been scared that he might not have covered his tracks well enough, he would be less frightened. Doug added that it would be more exciting too.

> A stolen apple always tastes sweeter.
>
> Doug, can you remember that first moment on the climbing wall when you placed your first handhold? What was it like as you looked up at the wall above you?

Doug laughed.

> I didn't look up, just as I didn't look down!
>
> Well, that fits perfectly with what I am wondering. Can I tell you what it is?

Wilbur looked vaguely interested, which was good enough for me.

> Doug, are you saying that even although you were being extremely brave, you still felt fear?
>
> I certainly did!
>
> And would you say that the fear was any less than it had been in the past?

Doug concluded that it was perhaps even greater.

> So, Doug, do you think it's possible that bravery may have nothing to do with getting rid of fear?

While Doug was considering his response, Wilbur chimed in.

> Yes, but the fear does get less because I got less scared the more I was a warrior.

I next spoke to Doug.

> Doug, do you think it's possible that, while no one in the world would wish a burglary on anyone, the burglary has been a bit of a bravery test? Anyone I have spoken to who has experienced a burglary says it really shook them up, and that they certainly felt frightened. However, do you think that Wilbur's bravery passed the test because even although the burglary shook him up it didn't shake the bravery out of him altogether?

Doug leapt on this idea with the full weight of his love for his son.

> Absolutely! I don't know if Wilbur's noticed this, but he has been getting braver at rugby. Even though he might not think so, I was impressed with the run he had last weekend and he scored a try at practice. And there was a point not long ago, just after the burglary, when he was going to give up rugby. I said he couldn't pull out. I told him that he needed to stay in the team for a season. To his credit, Wilbur stayed in there. He used his bravery and the freaky feelings got cut off at the pass.
>
> Wilbur, do you agree with your dad, that even though the burglary brought some of the freaky feelings back into your life, you used your bravery to stop them from becoming as powerful as they might have been?
>
> "Yeah," said Wilbur, looking at his father and then saying characteristically: "Dad, is it time to go now?"

Wilbur always seemed to be a better judge than either Doug or I when enough had been said.

A few weeks later I received an email from Liz.

> Thanks so much, Kay, we are so appreciative of the work you have done with Wilbur. The burglar worries seemed to have fallen away altogether. Not only that, but Wilbur went in a guitar competition on the weekend for the New Zealand Modern School of Music. He went into three different components of the competition. He got two gold and one bronze medal and won the trophy for the best guitar player in Wellington for his age group. His confidence is on a high... For the first time in ages, he is letting us take photos of him (with his medals, of course). Wilbur is in such an amazing space at the moment, we're not sure if he needs to see you again.
>
> Liz

As with most of the young people I meet, and especially those who have touched me the most or who I find most remarkable, thoughts of Wilbur would flit across my mind, and I would wonder how he was getting on. Had anorexia returned? I hardly dared to entertain the thought. Then, with some trepidation in September 2015, I emailed to Liz and Doug to ask if I could write about Wilbur and our work together and, of course, asked for news of their son.

This is an extract from Liz's email which I read with both relief and delight:

> Hi Kay,
> Lovely to hear from you. I hope that you are well. Wilbur is in such a good space at the moment! It's unbelievable! We have had a few hiccoughs over the years which may be to do with a surprising amount of stress in the family that he seems to be very sensitive to, but he is doing just great. His self-esteem has improved no end through music and sport. He does soccer and cricket. He now plays five instruments and is in three bands - one of them he put together and manages personally. Music is his life, really. He also got runner-up in his class last year for academic performance. As a family we don't emphasise academic performance at this age, but I thought I would let you know!

Notes

1 Ben Matulino and Simon Mannering are New Zealand rugby players.
2 Adrenalin Forest is an adventure theme park in Wellington.

Chapter 3
MOTHER APPRECIATION PARTIES

David Epston

Julie, despite her age of 40 or so, looked as if she was weary with life itself. At our first meeting, she immediately set about telling me what she considered to be the back story to her son Brandon's tantrums Brandon was 14. Julie met and married Brandon's Kiwi father overseas and the couple emigrated to New Zealand to make a home there. He was an international businessman whose travels took him away from New Zealand for various periods of time. From the very beginning of their marriage and more so after Brandon's birth, Julie's husband would scream at, revile, and beat her if his whims or demands were not urgently attended to. The beatings were frequent and often led to injuries requiring medical treatment. However, Julie was tolerant of this abuse because of her fervent desire for her son to grow up having a father, and she thought there was nothing she couldn't endure to see this longing come to pass. During her husband's absences overseas, Julie was determined to devote herself to her only child, doing everything imaginable to foster his initiative. When her husband returned to New Zealand, she noted how Brandon would withdraw into what she referred to as "a kind of hiding himself away." Brandon did agree when I asked if he had, in a manner of speaking, led two lives, one under his mother's care and another during his father's periods at home. As I might have expected, mother and son looked very kindly towards one another throughout this discussion.

However, Brandon went on the alert when Julie said that when he turned 11, he, as she put it, "started having a mind of his own." He no longer obeyed his father's commands as he had once been willing to do, and his father started to focus on and chastise him for every perceived breach of his orders. According to Julie, she did everything in her power to deflect her husband's attentions away from Brandon. No matter how hard she tried, however, she could not be successful for long and her husband would threaten her:

> Stay out of this. It's got nothing to do with you!

As Julie dreaded, her husband started to beat Brandon. This became unbearable to her, given her devotion to her son, especially when she observed how he had started "going into hiding all the time, even when his father was overseas." Despite her desire for her son to be raised by a father, she finally decided the violence her son was suffering was unconscionable and fled to a women's refuge during one of her husband's overseas trips. Again, as I might have expected, mother and son looked very kindly towards one another throughout this discussion.

This was soon to change dramatically. As Julie proceeded, her direct and forceful manner of speaking was replaced by a hesitance as if taking pains not to offend Brandon. She seemed to be checking with him after almost every carefully enunciated word. I was soon to learn she had good reason for such caution. Julie told me that since they started living on their own, Brandon had commenced screaming at, reviling, and beating her if any of his whims or demands was not attended to immediately. In fact,

> He calls me exactly the same names his father did!

Perhaps I was so taken aback by what Julie was sharing that I was no longer keeping an eye on Brandon when he erupted, screaming with such intensity that my first thought was for other families and their children in adjoining therapy rooms. I jumped out of my seat and rushed to him.

> Quick, give me your hand! This is an emergency! You are frightening the young children in the other therapy rooms!

Caught off guard, Brandon temporarily desisted from screaming, and allowed me to take his hand in mine.

> "You are going to be okay! Just slow your breathing and count down after me ... 10 ... 9 ... 8" and so on.

There were long pauses between each number. The boy recovered his equanimity and reassured me that we could proceed.

Julie, watching Brandon out of the corner of her eye, said that events such as I had just witnessed occurred between 10 and 15 times a day, whenever he disagreed with anything she said, or in response to any requests put to him. The disheartened look on her face, which for good reason she didn't dare to speak aloud, suggested several inquiries she may very well have embarked upon.

> Is this my fate? Was every beating I endured to provide Brandon with a father and every beating I accepted, to cover up for him, for nothing?

There were four more incidents of uncontrollable screaming when Brandon was affronted by a comment from his mother, each of which I was able to deal with by some version of my "emergency responding." Julie also mentioned her policy to which she had always been faithful:

> I decided to never say a bad word to Brandon about his father!

I turned to Brandon and asked if he could "bear the weight" of learning "the truth about your mother, even if her truth might be very different from your father's truth?" Wondering what was coming next, he tentatively agreed. Knowing the risks that we all were taking and constantly seeking Brandon's consent to proceed with further inquiry, I interviewed Julie about how she "would find ways to take the blows that were intended for Brandon, so he got off scot-free."

I carefully observed that Brandon listened intently and without comment. After a detailed account of several incidents, I turned to Brandon and asked:

> Did you have any idea before now that your mother went to such lengths to take the blows that otherwise would have fallen on you?

He admitted that this was entirely new to him.

> Do you mind telling me if knowing this changes your mind about the kind of mother you have?

He seemed to me somewhat ashamed to admit that it definitely had. I asked:

> Would you be willing to tell me what kind of mother you thought you had before knowing her 'truth'?

Before he could answer, I quickly turned to Julie and asked if she would allow him to tell his "truth" to her and "not think unkindly of him." She gave her consent to go ahead:

> Say what you really think. Don't worry, Brandon! I had to keep it from you!

Brandon shamefacedly said that he had thought his mother was "just plain dumb."

> Has your mother's 'truth' made you have second thoughts about your mother's stupidity?

He nodded ignominiously.

> Julie, did you play dumb so Brandon could go unharmed?

She admitted to having done so.

Although I will not detail the "temper tantrum party approach" (1) here, Brandon readily engaged in not only considering it but commissioning me to proceed with its introduction to him without delay. My guess is that it did not matter that I offered his mother "a double-your-money guarantee if he ever has another tantrum after leaving this building." What I recall vividly was his response to the requirements for his mother to either record or videotape a tantrum for his "temper tantrum party" to be attended by his best friends who he vowed to invite. Brandon resolutely informed his mother:

> Save your money on buying batteries!

He assured her:

> I will never have another tantrum as long as I live!

Julie stared at him in disbelief. I smiled to myself with a certain measure of confidence.

When they returned in a few weeks' time, Brandon had indeed lived up to his vow. Not surprisingly, we reviewed how he had gone from 10 to 15 tantrums a day, all of which bore a remarkable resemblance to his father's tantruming, to none. His mother referred to this turn of events as "having my son back again. I thought I had lost him forever!" She wept with joy and Brandon was far more at ease with himself and our company. I was able to relax my vigilance of him.

We once again discussed how Brandon had been able to understand the extent to which his mother had suffered to secure more than adequate care and protection for him. We talked, too, about how Julie had reached a point of such despair with his tantruming that she admitted to considering desperate measures such as seeking institutional care. When I inquired, Brandon willingly acknowledged that he was deeply concerned for his mother's well-being, although until he had found out her "truth," he conceded that he had taken her care and concern for granted. He had never considered her as sacrificing herself on his behalf but merely doing her duty. When Julie reassured me that she had a sense that I deeply appreciated her sacrifices on behalf of Brandon, I sought her permission to speak with him "privately," then adding "and secretly." I negotiated a pact of qualified secrecy with them both—"secrecy only for the time being." I added a rider to this and directed my comments to Julie:

> I give you my word of honor that in due course absolutely everything Brandon and I secretly discuss will be completely revealed to you!

This introduced an element of intrigue, if Brandon's furrowed brows were anything to go by as he, as yet, had no idea what in the world we would be keeping secret. Bemused but grinning, Julie readily gave her consent for us to proceed and hastily left us behind on her way to the waiting room.

> Brandon, do you mind drawing your chair closer to me? And do you mind if I draw my chair closer to you?

I looked at him kindly and asked:

> Are you worried about your mother's well-being?

He agreed.

> Have you come up with anything off your own bat to provide relief for her distress?

In fact, he had instituted some remedial action.

> Do you think your cups of tea are giving your mother sufficient relief for her to be entirely relieved of her distress?

Brandon conceded that the cups of tea weren't as effective as he had hoped. I then changed the subject from the inadequacy of his remedy with a very enthusiastically stated proposal for our consideration:

> By the way, have you ever heard of a surprise mother appreciation party?

Unsurprisingly, he readily acknowledged having never heard of such an event. But he did know something about the concept of a "surprise party."

From the outset of this conversation, I found myself regularly appending to every line of inquiry:

> If we do not keep it a secret, how can it be a surprise?

I asked Brandon if he might forego his current remedy on behalf of his mother's well-being and instead be willing to consider a "surprise mother appreciation party." He expressed considerable interest in what such an event might promise, even without yet knowing specific details.

> Have you ever been to a party?

Mother Appreciation Parties

Brandon recalled his attendances at various parties.

> Do you know a fair bit about parties in general even if you are still in the dark about 'surprise mother appreciation parties?' What do you think goes into having an ordinary, everyday party?

We came up with invitations and guests, food and drink, and usually something to celebrate like Easter, Christmas, or a birthday. We then set about figuring out the guest list before writing up the invitation.

> Who do you think you would like to invite to come to the surprise party to appreciate your mother as a wonderful mother? Who do you think would want to show her their appreciation for all the sacrifices she has made to ensure your care and protection?

Aunty Jenny stood out as one who was a strong advocate for Julie and assisted her in her flight and re-housing.

> Do you think you could secretly contact Aunty Jenny and find out if she'll come?

By the end of this meeting, we had a list of invitees whom Brandon promised to "secretly" contact between sessions.

At our next meeting, once again "private and secret," which meant Julie was excluded for most of it, I was not surprised to learn that Aunty Jenny and Julie's best friend, Beth, a former neighbor, had insisted on assisting Brandon with the preparations. Brandon had already come up with a list proposing the food and drinks and how Aunty Jenny and Beth were organizing that along the lines of "bring a drink and a plate of food to share." Brandon reported considerable momentum towards the scheduled date that they had agreed on.

> By the way, Brandon, how are you doing keeping the 'mother appreciation party' secret so it will turn to be a surprise?

Brandon chuckled with pleasurable mischief, telling me about the subterfuges he had gotten up to avoid detection. I suspected Julie knew something was up but was allowing him free rein here. Conspiring together like this had allowed Brandon and me to draw closer, and by now we were entirely at ease with one another.

Still, I had some reservations about my next question:

> I suppose you have been wondering how you go about 'appreciating a mother' at a surprise mother appreciation party?

He admitted that he "didn't have a clue."
What interested me was that Brandon then asked if I had any ideas.

> I have, but you might be surprised by what a son your age gets up to.

He cautiously urged me to proceed.

> Well, the only way I know how you can show your appreciation of your mother at her surprise party is by giving a 'mother appreciation speech'!

The fact that he was speechless gave me sufficient time to add:

> Hey, don't worry about it! It will be easier than you think. I will ask your mother appreciation questions and you will reply with mother appreciation answers. And as we go along, I will take notes and type it up as your speech. You might even give it to your mom afterwards so she can keep it with your baby photographs and other stuff she keeps as memories.

We agreed on another appointment to have all the time we required to "write a speech your mother will never forget as long as she lives."

We summoned Julie into the room and sought her permission for one more private and secret meeting. Julie said that would be fine. She laughed, telling us:

> You can have as many secret meetings as you guys need. Brandon has become so much more willing to help me around the house and accept my rules. Whatever you guys are doing secretly is working!

We winked at one another, still retaining our resolve to ensure it would be a

> surprise mother appreciation party.

In addition to preparing Brandon's "mother appreciation speech," we also discussed how we might ensure the event was a "surprise party." Brandon cooked up the idea of having Aunty Jenny take his mother to an early movie. He and Beth would make sure all the guests arrived before they returned home and were out of sight. Their cars would be parked around the block so as not to alert Julie. All the guests would ready themselves to surprise Julie as she entered her home.

I have never attended such a celebration in person, but I couldn't wait to hear from Brandon, who promised to phone me "first thing" the day after the surprise party. I heard it went well and Julie agreed when, at my request, he called her to the phone. I asked:

Was it a surprise?

Julie said the party was the best surprise she had ever had. I invited mother and son to meet one more time to tell me all about it. That was my first post-party meeting and, along with others similar, it became one of the most memorable events of my professional career.

The highlight of the post-party meeting was Brandon agreeing, at my request, to re-read his "surprise mother appreciation speech" aloud to me in Julie's presence. He asked his mother for it, and she produced it from her purse, sealed in a plastic bag. She handed the document over like a person from a persecuted religion showing a relic in secret to a coreligionist. I asked if Brandon might stand up and face his mother. Once again, I am sure they were looking kindly towards one another. He hesitated, clearing his throat before he began.

> To everyone here, I want you to know why I planned and with Aunty Jenny and Beth's help organised a surprise mother appreciation party for my mom. I am so grateful to her doing everything she could to make sure of my care and protection. Most of you know that my father would scream at my mother, call her terrible names, and beat her up for just about anything. She had to follow his orders, and if she didn't so something he ordered perfectly or right away, that was the reason he would give for hurting and beating her, sometimes injuring her.
>
> I was so scared, but she always made sure I was safe and hidden away in my room. When he was overseas, I now realise she did everything she could to make me believe in myself. She said that I hid myself away when Dad lived

81

with us, and I guess she was trying to have me come out of myself when he wasn't at home. Perhaps she knew what was coming when I got older and didn't always do everything right away when my father ordered me around. Then he started screaming at me and calling me names. And it wasn't too long before he beat me up too, even if it wasn't as bad as what Mom got. Then my mom started getting stupid. Or at least that is what I thought at the time. She would do really obvious things that would get her a beating when it was me who was at fault. Like the time I ate all the ice cream not knowing my father would come home on an earlier flight. And my father had to have ice cream for pudding or else. I told Mom what I had done, and she just smiled and told me to stay in my room. I heard my father screaming, and Mom said that it was her fault and that she had wanted to eat some ice cream. This made him scream louder and hurt her more. She kept doing lots of stupid things like this.

Just a month or more ago, Mom told me she did it on purpose to keep me safe. I was ashamed as, after we lived at the women's refuge and then got this apartment, I started screaming and calling Mom the same names Dad did. I hit her too. One reason for my speech is to tell you how ashamed I am and how I want Mom to know how much I respect her for saving me from my father's violence. She suffered so I would not suffer. Now, can anyone here think of a better reason for a son my age to hold a surprise party to appreciate his mother? When I am older and maybe have a son of my own, I hope my mother will be as wonderful to him as she is to me. Can everyone take a glass of something and can we sing 'For she's a jolly good mother!'

I didn't ask what had happened to those attending the party witnessing Brandon's change of heart, but at the post-party reading, all of us had to dry the tears from our eyes. They shared memories of the fun everyone had, especially Julie. As he had promised me, Brandon had seen to it that she didn't do a lick of work at her party.

Suggested Reading

Epston, D. (1992). Temper tantrum parties: Saving face, losing face, or going off your face? In Epston, D. & White, M. (Eds.), *Experience, contradiction, narrative and imagination* (pp. 37-74). Adelaide: Dulwich Centre Publications.

Epston, D., Lobovits, D., & Freeman, J., introduction by Murphy, S. (2008). Annals of the new Dave: Status—abled, disabled or weirdly-abled? In Epston, D. (Ed.), *Down under and up over: Travels with narrative therapy* (pp. 41-60). Warrington: Association of Family Therapy. A free copy of this book will be sent to anyone applying to dejbftc@xtra.co.nz for PDFs of the hard copy version. I thank the Association of Family Therapy (UK) for allowing me to distribute it in this fashion.

See Maisel, R., Epston, D., & Borden, A. (2004). *Biting the hand that starves you: Inspiring resistance to anorexia/bulimia.* New York: W.W. Norton; Epston, D., & Maisel, R. (2009). Anti-anorexia/bulimia: A polemics of life and death. In Malson, H. & Burns, M. (Eds.), *Critical feminist approaches to dis/orders* (pp. 209-220). London: Routledge; Epston, D. (1999). *Co-research—The making of an alternative knowledge.* Retrieved from http://www.narrativeapproaches. com/antianorexia%20folder/anti_anorexia_index.htm; Lock, A., Epston, D., & Maisel, R. (2004). Countering that which is called anorexia. *Narrative Inquiry, 14*(2), 275-302; Lock, A., Epston, D., & Maisel, R. (2005). Resisting anorexia/ bulimia: Foucauldian perspectives in narrative therapy. *Journal of Guidance and Counselling, 33*(3), 315-332.

Chapter 4

"A NEW SURPRISE OF EXISTING: THE LAST THING I EVER WAS – WAS SILENT"

A Poetic Response to Patriarchal Malice

JOYFULLY CO-AUTHORED BY SANNI PALJAKKA AND FABIOLA

Dear Reader,
Please consider a heads-up to this account: I compose poems[1] after each therapy conversation to capture significant expressions and discoveries that stood out to me. Consequently, I read the poems aloud to my clients at the beginning of our next meeting, and we often refer back to them as part and parcel of our conversations. I ask you as readers to allow me to weave in and out of these poems freely as I would with my clients, and to consider them, not as surplus summaries, but as integral and substantive forces to drive the Narrative and its work forward. At the outset of each chapter, I provide hints to some of the more dramatic turns in my conversations with Fabiola by way of dialogue and then present the poem written afterwards.
I invite you to take up these hints and look inside each of the poems represented in this account for the manner in which these turning points were inscribed into the poems.

Chapter 1: Why Me?

"Why me?" Fabiola asked on the fine spring day when I ventured the proposal to co-author this book chapter together. I had told her that she was the person that came immediately to my mind as I was rather hesitantly surveying this writing project. "Why me?" I knew my response to this question mattered, not because I felt any inclination to convince her of the idea of writing about her life, but because this exchange was a chance to be a witness to her life. I told her the obvious reason first:

> Well, because I know you are interested in writing and doing this together might not be too mind-numbing or tiresome for you....

Fabiola nodded, and I went on:

> But also, how do I say this, Fabiola? Your story is strong! Do you know when I first started working here, I had serious questions whether I could be of any use to people who have experienced serious mistreatment. I wondered what on earth I could do. But your story is strong and clear that 'discernments' between love and mistreatment are possible, and together, we can find the means to tell of these discernments. The things you have told me here, Fabiola, are worthy of attention for other therapists, and maybe even encouraging of them to look again at what women are saying in the aftermath of such experiences. Remember how you talked about 'leaving behind his petty arena to free your imagination and to explore all of New York....'. I want to tell everyone that you said that, and what you meant by it, and that you THEN went ahead to DO that! I think it might inspire other therapists to start looking for ways in which women don't just simply protest their mistreatment but, in fact, go ahead to create lives full of freedom of imagination! Maybe telling this story could shore them up to do this work without limiting their imaginations either!

Fabiola laughed at my explanation and then told a story of a speech she had recently prepared and delivered that had touched on parts of her personal experiences of abuse and how the group of women had responded with a standing ovation.

"I wonder, Fabiola, what would move an audience to rise to their feet?" I asked.

I think they recognized how deeply I dug...I think they are inspired by someone's commitment to growth.

I smiled and inquired further:

Growth? Here is this word again that you have been using so often to describe what you have been trying for. Can you help me understand this word growth better? If you follow it, where does it take your life?

Fabiola was thoughtful.

It expands my life.
Oh, I see. Are you saying that perhaps the audience saw what I saw, your steadfast refusal of the efforts to shrink your life and always responding with an expansion in all the moments when the chips were down?
Yes. Maybe. I think that is what they recognised.
And in recognition of your talent at expansion, they rose to their feet? Did they amplify your efforts at expansion?

Fabiola smiled at the thought.

Hey, I am remembering about the word amplification, that it is the call of a witness to amplify the words of another... And I am also remembering a line from a poem that says that love is the amplification of another. What do think of this Fabiola?
That sounds nice to think of the audience that way.

Below is my poetic version of what Fabiola had told me:

I composed and read my story
to a standing ovation
and what is in my story
that makes others rise to it?
I saw it and I wondered.

I dug really deeply
into my obsession with growth
and its deepening and widening powers

> my voice and my freedom
> stand for an expansion
> -love
> is an amplification
> of another?

Fabiola and I have often wondered out loud what love is. If love is an "expansion" or an "amplification," as the poem says, then my quest is, above all other considerations, to amplify Fabiola's voice and knowing.

CHAPTER 2: THE FRESHNESS OF OUR BEGINNING

Fabiola and I first met six months earlier on a cold November day after her referral to me by another therapist. The change of therapists had happened rather suddenly and jaggedly. Fabiola came to meet me with questions about the idea of "beginning again" with a stranger and a sense of wariness of spending time and effort to reiterate what had been meaningful to her in her previous therapy. We considered the option of me approaching her previous therapist for a written summary, as a point of reference that we could review, to ease the burden of catching me up. Fabiola was not sure of this idea and grew tearful, overwhelmed by being "thrown into this new relationship" and the pressure she felt to find a "good beginning."

Honorably, she fought for her words to let me in on this struggle.

> This is the first new relationship I am getting into now at the end of a difficult three years. It is all unknown and I am not sure how to feel. Is this what it is like to get into a new relationship?
>
> I guess it is! The one thing I know for sure is that no one makes the decision to come here *lightly*. I have come to know something about what it takes for people to make this appointment and *keep* it, when I know there are a hundred other more enjoyable things to do on a cold Wednesday night, like spending the evening with Netflix or with tea or wine. So, this always has me thinking that there must be something that really matters, something that is really significant that is currently happening to you, in your life, for you to come here tonight to begin again with me, another stranger? Is this right?
>
> There are things that really matter to me! I just don't know where to begin....

Fabiola's voice broke as an accusation against her person formed.

> Maybe I am not able to trust people. Maybe this is too hard, and I should just go....

I fought for words as well and asked:

> Or maybe your trust is precious?

I was feeling a rush of respect towards Fabiola's struggle and her honesty with me. I could not help wondering if I was already experiencing the practice of her trust in me, but I was offended on her behalf that her efforts were being sullied by such an explanation.

I thought highly of her refusal of the usual politeness of first meetings to address me so candidly. I also strongly suspected that if she were to leave now, the accusation that she is just not able to trust people and the feelings of failure might set upon her life and person like concrete. Whatever else, I did not want her to depart thinking she had failed! In the therapeutic code that conspires against people, "the ability to trust" has been entirely co-opted to serve as but one powerful starting point to construct oneself as a broken or failed self. Fabiola didn't answer, but became tearful, so I proceeded softly:

> Fabiola, there have been many others who have sat where you sit now and have told me that they are failing at trust. I have concluded that if we have nothing else to make a woman feel like shit about themselves, then that accusation invariably works.

Fabiola smiled a little at me.

> They have told me that I trust too easily and then they have told me that I don't trust enough.

I smiled back.

> Oh great, equal opportunity failure for a woman in a shitty circumstance, hey? No way to get it right; that's awesome.

She smiled again. Fortified, I went on:

> And I *am* a stranger, and say, your trust was indeed precious, how would you know whether I am worthy of your trust?

Fabiola and I came to a rather odd conclusion: we agreed to suspend any therapeutic ventures in favor of an experiment with new beginnings.

> How about we don't do any "therapisty" stuff at all. Since you already walked here and it is kind of cold and shitty out, how about I just tell you a little bit about myself for the time that remains?

Fabiola agreed with relief.

> I'll tell you a little about what other women have asked me in their attempts to discern my trustworthiness and then you might invent some questions of your own to add.

In the impromptu introduction that followed, I spoke about what Narrative Therapy means to me, about my accent, my move to Canada and the first time I had seen the prairie. Fabiola suddenly interrupted and asserted herself:

> You know what. I came in here feeling so unsafe, so agitated. I don't know why my previous therapist didn't catch you up. But I am not angry or disappointed now. You know what! Don't bother contacting her. I have a voice! Maybe this is an opportunity for freedom, to embark on this on my own, to define myself, to reinvent myself. I know what you meant by how moved you were about the prairie. I have taken a road trip through the prairies too, and what you said reinforced my curiosity about my own trip....

I was surprised to say the least.

> What? What happened, Fabiola, as you were listening to me? Did you come to some discernment about trust, or your voice, or the prairies? I don't even know what happened just now?

She smiled at me and explained.

> You shared more deeply than I thought you would. I thought you would just talk about your professional training. But you went beyond that. And I connected with what you said about being away from home, and then I thought about the freedom I felt when I left home and what it was like to return to the prairie. And it made me curious about this new freedom that we have to talk about together now. Look, the only thing you really need to know is that I broke up with my boyfriend three years ago. He had a difficult past, and anyway, he didn't take well to the break-up. He harassed me, smeared me, threatened me, broke my car windows, followed me to work and to my house. He has been unrelenting for the past three years, his various attempts to hurt me and scare me, and now there is a Restraining Order in place since

this summer. I am actually quite finished with all of this, and I have recently decided not to hear any more news about him, I've asked my colleagues and friends to shield me from any more news. You know what, I want a new beginning in my life and with you. I want all the freshness of my new beginning away from his efforts to smear me.

"So here it is!" I said.

Did you somehow travel from a space of no words to the freedom of your own words? To the 'freshness of a new beginning', no less?

We smiled at each other.
Our session was finished, but I couldn't resist one more comment:

Hey Fabiola, you said at the beginning that maybe you suck at trust. Can you tell me again what you just did and thought in practicing trust with me?

She thought a while and said:

I considered leaving, you know, just walking out of here. But when you offered to become less of stranger to me, I told myself to sit. 'Just give it a chance', I told myself, 'just listen and see.'

It was my turn to smile.

Did you just give me both the very definition of trust and a real-life example of what it takes to give a stranger the preciousness of your trust: 'just give it a chance, just listen and see.' Is this what trust sounds like in action?

Fabiola ventured:

Well, maybe this was an *activated kind of* trust today.

Only one thing was certain: we parted somehow other than wary strangers, and a poem of our words on this day was born:

The Freshness of My New Beginning

As I am entering into a new place
There is strangeness here
And I think of safety and trust
And I wonder:
Is this what it is like to get into a new relationship,
Is this what that feels like?

Don't give me old news
Of my difficult 3 years
Of harassment and smear campaigns and threats
And break-ins into my person
I closed the door
And put a sign up: Return to Sender.

And now I think of the freedom
To reinvent myself
Who am I becoming
Without the notes
Of my past fluttering in
Or the mailbox clanking at every hour:
I have a voice!
And this is an opportunity for freedom to define myself
As other than what I was made
Or threatened or written to be.

I find myself thinking:
Just give it a chance,
Just listen and see.
And I wonder:
Is this the activated start of trust
That I have only just remembered in this
Fresh prairie space?
Is this a trust that grows
The beauty of a prairie
And the excitement of a road trip
Through the scenery I once knew
And now have the freedom to know anew?

Chapter 3: I Am the Girl with the Voice of Resolve

When Fabiola returned to my office two weeks later, I read the above-mentioned poem to her. She was visibly moved and exclaimed:

> That was so unexpected!

I laughed.

> *What* was unexpected?
> "My voice! I can hear it!" she declared.
> Right, it says so right here in the poem, '*I have a voice!*' What did your voice sound like to you just now when I read this to you?
> It sounds firm. It's really clear. You know sometimes things happen that muffle the sounds from within, but I know there is a voice that comes from within and I can listen to it, and can operate from it and it's really clear.

I couldn't resist another question.

> Fabiola, tell me how to write about that in my next note to you. Shall I write 'firm voice' or 'clear voice,' or what kind of a voice is this voice of yours? What is its quality?

Fabiola offered:

> It's a resolved voice! That's what it sounds like to me.
> A resolved voice, alright, a voice of resolve! I get it! And there have been quite the attempts to muffle your voice in the past few years, with your ex trying to muffle it. Am I right in thinking that? ... That must be quite the voice of resolve! Can you tell me how your voice resolved to come through in spite of the muffling? How might you say that?

Here is my poetic reflection of this part of the conversation:

> against the attempts
> to muffle the sounds from within
> my voice of resolve
> comes through

> I listen,
> and it is really firm
>
> I know that his betrayal of my trust is his;
>
> but I needed my firm voice
> to say this over and over:
> I said it to coworkers: "please shield me"
> I said it to the police: "please protect me"
> and I said it in court,
> right next to my ineffective lawyer
> "please stop him."

In the above exchange I found out how Fabiola had come to rely on "her voice of resolve" in coming through in formidable circumstances with her coworkers, the police, and in court seeking protection against her ex-boyfriend's harassment, stalking and threats against her person. It had not started out this way. Fabiola said that when her ex-boyfriend first started publishing stories of her on social media after their break-up and started to come by at her place of work to yell and rage at her, she had felt guilty, embarrassed and anxious. She was unable to respond, searching her mind all day and night what she had done wrong and whether she had had a right to ask for a separation or owed him more time and care.

I interrupted

> Hold on. *Owed* him? Whose idea is that, Fabiola? Is someone telling you that you owed him more time and care?

Fabiola looked bemused considering my question.

> That's funny. I didn't realise that. *He* says that. That's what he always says. Whenever he comes to my work, he yells that I owe him a conversation.

I inquired:

> What do you think of that idea that you owe him something?

> I did talk to him. We talked on the phone quite a few times when I broke up with him. I wrote out my thoughts too and explained to him why I wanted out. I actually waited to tell him. I waited to make sure that I was sure. He just didn't want to accept the break-up.

I seized upon this.

> Fabiola, this is important, especially if this question has kept you up at night. And you might not be surprised to know that I happen to meet with a lot of people who are in the midst of a break-up, whether they are the one instigating the leaving or bearing the leaving. Tell me on their behalf as well, what do we owe each other as human beings during a break-up? Or what are the ethics of a break-up for the leaver as well as the one who is left?
>
> Actually, I think that I'm okay with how I went about it. I think it's good to have a conversation and tell a person why it's over. And it's okay to try and be sure but kind about it....

Earnestly, and in hopes of underscoring the significance of her words, I asked:

> If I told others who are in the midst of a break-up how you went about this, about how you held yourself to a moral code of speaking your decision to the person, and speaking it clearly and kindly, would I be capturing your moral code correctly?
>
> Yes! I would say so. But he still continues to demand something of me, that I still owe him....
>
> I see. Are there some words you have for people who are being left, who are in the midst of that heartbreak? How ought we as humans respond morally to the end of love, especially perhaps when we didn't wish for it to come to an end?

Fabiola was deep in thought. Breaking from it, she then spoke softly about the struggles her ex-boyfriend had been up against in his life and her understanding of how it came to be that he granted himself permission to refuse her right to end the relationship.

> I wonder, Fabiola, whether his refusal of your rights is being backed up by some ideas out there that we as women somehow owe our continued

presence, our love, our care to men? Is it possible that there are ideas out there that help men to give themselves permission to dismiss our rights, our decisions, and especially our 'no's' to them?

Fabiola deliberated on this question. I went on, softly:

And how is it that your voice, nevertheless, has been so clear in the face of his powerful refusals, that your voice has so clearly and formidably insisted on your rights with your coworkers, with the police, and in court?

Fabiola spoke of the clarity of her own moral considerations in the face of his attacks on her person that grew more fearsome over time. She described incidents in which her coworkers hid her in closets at work when he came around, and how she found her car windows shattered on more than one occasion. Her ex also started publishing veritable facsimiles of 'Wanted' posters in her neighborhood by her house, complete with a photograph of her and an outline of how horrible a person she was. These posters and stickers also appeared nearby her parents' house. Fabiola eloquently described what it was like to drive through the neighborhood to and from work trying to keep her eyes fixed on the road in front of her.

Fabiola's parents and friends were supportive but started wondering what she had done to invite this kind of hatred, speculating as to whether her "boundaries" were too "soft" for her to discern between trustworthy and untrustworthy romantic partners. In light of these questions and doubts and his formidable expressions of entitlement to her presence in his life, her statement of "I know that his betrayal of my trust is his" was hard won. In addition, her actions of speaking to the police and in the court seeking a Restraining Order have to be considered accomplishments of discernment and clarity regarding Fabiola's moral code for people's treatment of each other in the wake of a painful separation. Fabiola had successfully defended her right to safety of her mind and her person, and the court had subsequently granted her a Restraining Order!

I have come to know something of what it takes for women to go to the police, or tell their story of mistreatment in court, over the years at my therapy office. I knew immediately that this was no ordinary feat of resolve and clarity on Fabiola's part. I also had a hunch that for her "voice" to show up like this on her behalf to accompany and counsel her toward moral resolve through a formidably vulnerable time, it likely had a rather interesting history. And yet I listened to her characterizing herself quite differently. *"I never had a voice like this before. I was always just quiet. I never spoke up to anyone. I never stood up for myself like this..."* I was offended on Fabiola's behalf yet again, that some story of *"quietness"* or *"soft-boundaried-ness"* had downgraded her ethical accomplishments here and had left her bereft of a possible substantive counterhistory of her actions.

We were about to cast her recent actions as merely singular and insignificant accidents, undertaken to lessen her embarrassment about choosing an untrustworthy partner, and her supposed presumptive guilt over the vicious turn the break-up had taken.

I took a breath and hazarded to inquire:

> I wonder about that Fabiola. If your voice showed up so powerfully now, that it quite literally took on a 'leadership role', as you say in your life over the past couple years, forgive me but I can't help but wonder whether you've heard it before at different turning points in your life? Do you remember if your voice has come to your aid before? Has it accompanied you through difficult experiences before? Do you remember it being there, like a friend to you of sorts, speaking to you about who you are and what you can do? I don't know....

Fabiola was again deep in thought. And then I literally "saw" her recall a vivid memory in the brightening of the expression on her face. She remembered how she had broken her "quietness'" in acts of protection for her younger brother growing up, and how clearly her voice had come to counsel her to leave her hometown as a young professional.

Here is my poetic reflection of Fabiola's sudden remembrance of a counterhistory of her voice:

> my voice has taken on a more significant role
> a leadership role as of late
> and suddenly I am reminded of
> its long history in my life.
>
> I remember how it counseled
> silence and light steps

around my mom's temper
- except when she tried to kick in the bathroom door
to get to my little brother.
"leave him alone"
my voice shouted
and the resolve in it was such
that she turned and walked away.

I remember how it stopped me in my tracks
in that moment on Stephen Avenue
in an epiphany of the ordinary
"it is time for you to leave Calgary."
- and the resolve in it was such
that it spawned my 15-year-old journey to Montreal Toronto and the US
and the experience of a rush of welcome freedom.

and when the ghosts came back
upon my return,
demanding their pound of flesh
they didn't quite know
that I am well trained
in the longing for freedom
the insistence on justice
the fight for a human's rights
and the knowing when something was wrong.
what the ghosts didn't know
is that
when I kicked those boys in the legs
and yelled for them to leave my brother alone
they too walked away.

I am the girl
with the inexorable soul
and the voice of resolve
that no show of pompous force
has daunted.

Chapter 4: My Voice Was Delivered To Me In a Box

Something quite extraordinary happened soon after our session exploring a history of Fabiola's voice. Fabiola immediately announced on her arrival:

> My dad surprised me and came to my house with a box of my journals that I had kept since I was 11 years old.

I wanted to know more.

> What do you mean your journals? A box of them? How many were there?
> 32.

"32!"
I laughed.

> I am trying to imagine what it would be like, Fabiola, to open the box? Tell me everything.

Fabiola smiled at me.

> I opened the box and the first one was from when I was 11. On the first page it said, 'This is my first diary.'

Fabiola went on to recount what she discovered on the pages of the journals she had written over the years and then declared:

> I realize I wasn't silent. The last thing I was, was silent.

I expect the poem that emerged from our conversations about the contents of this box require no further explanation from me:

> my voice was delivered to me in a box
> 2 weeks ago
> "this is my first diary" my 11-year-old wrote
> and I have been thinking ever since.

99

my existence is thanks to the words I wrote.
in my house of neglect and unreturned affections
I wrote me an existence
a home
a place that listened:
I managed to fill 32 journals
with my voice.
and looking at the books filled with my words
I realize that I wasn't silent
up against the daily fear and mom's temper
and the tiptoeing we had to do
and the counting of blinks when I tried to talk to her
about my days and what mattered to my little heart
the last thing I ever was, was silent.
I always craved a safe place
that wouldn't berate me
betray me
gloss over my sense of worth
even as I was talking.
and did I already then
know something about my own innocence
that was being trampled on every day?
and what did I know of love?
in my journals
I created a world in which
the blank page said to me
"say more, sweetheart"
"I want to know your stories, honey."
something has shifted
as of late
something precious has been returned to me:
perhaps it is an
A for astute
a B for bold
and a C for confident
- all the letters of an innocent
girl's writing
have come to intertwine with me as I am,

    a grown woman today.
    and they have begun
    to question
    the Ds for doubt
    and the Gs for guilt
    that gripped me all that time ago.

In the midst of Fabiola's rediscovery of her journals and the sound of her voice within them, she surprised me yet again. She returned to our next session with a piece of writing of her own, addressed to me, and written from her own living room among her journals that were strewn about like testaments of a new emergence. I am reprinting Fabiola's note to me in full for the reasons that it stands both as a reflection of the effects of my poetry-writing practice to my clients as well as an expansion of Fabiola's own thoughts about her discoveries in our work and in her life:

    In Reply to Your Conversation Summaries

    Dear Sanni,

    I was hit with emotion when I first heard you read your summary
    of our first conversation,
    unable to express sufficient thanks to you
    for fear that I would cry if I uttered anything at all.

    The first time I heard you read your summary of our first
    conversation,
    I felt an unfamiliar surprise of existing
    through hearing what I had expressed to you
    only two weeks prior,
    and then later, miraculously, in the form of a thoughtful poem.

    Beyond the emotions
    and the surprise,
    I felt a sensation of coming into shape
    through words, emotions, and thoughts that came from me
    but that I assumed had no previous form or place to go,

after they left me.
Until they returned to me again,
with a permanent home
in your touching reflective poem.

Like a pool of water stagnating into dryness,
the particles lifted themselves up to take shape into something
plentiful and rhythmic.
Like a broken object played in rewind,
the pieces picked themselves up to become something meaningful
and whole.

My spirit
now in your words
traveled
from my head, my heart
out of my mouth
onto the pages of your notebook
and then into your poem:
its final destination.

A destination
where I seemed to have a shape
where I seemed to have an identity
where I seemed to exist.

***

And yet,

as I witnessed my thoughts and emotions take up residence in your written words, Sanni,
I should not have been surprised,
not me,
not at all.

At the age of 11,
chance came to me with blank pages,

and without hesitating,
I followed its cue
filling those pages with words upon words
about my days, thoughts, worries,
filling those pages with words breathing stories about me.
Now, at the age of 43,
it is not chance but desire
that drives me to write about these things still,
with 32 journals?
filled page upon page with words
from then until now.

What did that young girl know
on that day when chance visited her?

Did she begin to write down words
to create a safe place where she would be heard
when she wanted to speak?
Did she already know that those words,
spoken in their familial space,
would find no willing ears,
no gentle understandings,
no affectionate returns?
Did she write down words
to retreat to a place where she could exist
without reproach,
without fear,
without rejection?

Beyond her written words,
that young girl was encouraged to be silent,
she was expected to be silent,
and she kept silent,
obediently and responsibly.

33 (?)journals filled from page to page
with word upon word

tell a different story:
that there was never silence,
that there is never silence in places
where there is anger, pain, fear, and neglect.

Did the act of writing by that young girl,
who was yearning to speak,
loudly,
yearning to be heard,
and desperately yearning to find a loving place in an unloving world,
save me from being silenced,
save me from being erased completely?

Beyond the 33 journals,
formlessness is what I have always known,
uncertainty about who I was,
confusion about how to exist among others,
discomfort around others,
thinking for others,
feeling responsible only for others,
for I have always been uttering the words of others.

***

In a world where I always stretched far beyond myself for others,
did I return to the written word to find and preserve my voice?
Did I return to it for easy love?
Did I return to it to connect with my purpose?
Did I return to it repeatedly for desperate freedom?

Have you, Sanni, with your soothing voice reaching me through our words in your summaries,
come into my life, like chance did 32 years ago, to confirm that this is where my fate lies: in the written word?

Chapter 5: My Soul Is Roaming

Fabiola returned in early January after a trip to New York. She told me how she had booked her trip out of a sudden longing to sit in a coffee shop and write in a journal, to walk "somewhere where things are big" and visit art galleries. She said that Christmastime was difficult for her ex-boyfriend, and that she had come to anticipate some kind of a renewed "eruption" of his and another attempt to capture her in his "petty arena" of attacks despite the Restraining Order that remained in place. I was full of questions.

> From the petty arena to where things are big, hey?

Smiling, she recounted:

> Yeah. I imagine that I would leave him behind in his own petty arena, to churn there and struggle against his own walls of petty malice. And I wouldn't be there at all. I'd be off, elsewhere.

I laughed in delight over her imagery, and asked excitedly:

> Like that game, Pacman, remember that? He's stuck in his own arena, his own limited labyrinth, chomping and churning and whatever Pacman does in his arena. Only you are long gone, not even in the game! Meanwhile *you* are in another world, in New York!

Fabiola laughed with me, her eyes shining more brightly than I had ever seen before. I pursued this:

> Well, tell me everything! This idea of yours has me so excited. Tell me what sparked it! What did you long to find where 'things are big', Fabiola? What did your soul long for when you booked the trip? Where does art and writing take your soul, Fabiola?

Fabiola said she didn't have anything particular in mind for her trip, except to "take her soul out" and let it "go where New York would take it."
    I couldn't resist.

From Pacman-arena to the Big Apple of all places, Fabiola.

Fabiola's laughter rang free. Then she went on to describe it this way;

> I have three years of heavy and dense material, Sanni. For three years I have lived in his petty arena, always defending myself, always expecting his next attack, always juggling anxiety and fear about his next move. It's been three years of damage control. But that is not what I am supposed to be doing with my life. If I keep shrinking myself and my life to just keep reacting to and protesting every little thing he does, what happens to me and my dreams? I would be letting him keep me small! 20 years from now, I don't want to wake up and realize that he captured all of my dreams of what my life can be and that I couldn't grow to be a bigger person in this time. I went to New York, Sanni, because I decided I am going to be as big a person as I can be. I wrote it on my chalkboard at home: Make this about something bigger, Fabiola.

On this snowy day, Fabiola taught me a lesson I will never forget. I ventured:

> Make this about something bigger indeed. I see. I see it, Fabiola. Restraining Orders might, if they work, keep a person 200 meters from another person, but what about the restraining orders needed for our souls? The restraining orders to keep smear stories and continued threats from stealing a person's imagination, dreams, future and relationships? Did you just accomplish what the Restraining Order couldn't? Did you order your soul to roam free into a big future too?

In this conversation, Fabiola's trip to New York took shape in front of both of us as a *pièce de résistance*. But her trip was not just a protest to her ex-boyfriend's mistreatment of her. It was also a living into her counter-history of a girl, then merely 11, with an inexorable soul and a voice of resolve who can tell love from unlove, give to another her precious trust, and protect herself and others when trust is broken, and whose longing for the bigness of the world resounds as vivaciously as ever. "I even went on a date while I was there, Sanni!" Fabiola exclaimed in this conversation with a smile of pride. The poem of this conversation was a pure pleasure to compose:

I took my soul out
For long walks
And to stand in front of art
And to write in coffee shops

I took my soul out
And let it go
wherever New York would take it.

I stepped out of his petty arena
And left him behind to hit his own walls

I stepped out and took my soul
To the Big Apple instead.
And to let the big world turn my head
And move me and expand me
Without knowing where we would end up.
And then I went on a date, if you can believe that.
And then I went on another.

Because I refuse to let my soul and my head
And my hopes and my imagination
Be captured
By the petty maliciousness I have known.
There are decent guys out there
And healthy relationships for me to step into
I am sure of it.

So don't think I am about to let another
Small arena
Intrude on my soul:
No, dad, I will not text you every day
And no, I will not search my body for whether
It happens to please the gaze of one man

My soul is roaming
To find her special way of loving
And becoming a beloved
And yes, please, let it be as free as all of the Empire State of Mind....

Chapter 6: Finally

After Fabiola decided to leave the petty arena of her ex-boyfriend's malice behind and engage with her big dreams for her future instead, her ex-boyfriend staged a few more formidable come-backs to reinstate his grip on her life. I reflected to her:

> If not tied to me by bounds of love, then by bounds of malice?

Fabiola nodded quietly and described how her ex had appeared at her workplace attempting to assault her, how he papered the parameters of a gathering space of a work-presentation she facilitated with his 'Wanted' circulars, how her bedroom windows were smashed at 2 am yet again, and how she saw his grainy image on the surveillance footage the morning after. She intoned quietly:

> What misery must his life be to have nothing better to do on a random night at 2 am.

As I wondered about her sense of calm, she remarked that worse than his continued "juvenile stunts" were the many invitations for her to perform some kind of proper "victim role."

"Juvenile stunts, Fabiola?", I asked.

> Now there's some words. Here he is thinking to draw you in to malice and terror, and here you are, downgrading his actions to the level of juvenile stunts. What does your choice of words here suggest about your position in regard to his attempt to dominate your life?
>
> His attempts are blunt endeavors to limit my life. I have been quite relaxed about it, and have done okay with responding, calmly calling the police each time. Actually, what has bothered me way more than his actions of late are some of the more sophisticated clippings of my wings that others have delivered to me.

Fabiola went on to describe some of these sophisticated clippings: the office gossip about her ex-boyfriend's recent appearance outside of her work, as well as the veiled accusations by the police that she did not appear to be struggling enough to warrant help, and her friends' encouragements to appear "weaker" in order to inspire the legal help and justice that she sought.

I interjected.

Weaker? Wow, there's a word. How about we appear a bit "weaker" in order to deserve help or justice. Is that how this goes?

Fabiola nodded.

Yes, my friends actually used the word "hysterical."

I raised my eyebrows mischievously and Fabiola responded:

They are trying to be helpful. They thought I should have cried more and been more hysterical in the meeting with the crown prosecutor and that I should have emphasised how afraid I am. That just didn't occur to me!

I was stunned by the clarity of this line of thinking.

Wow. Fuck, Fabiola, is it possible that your friends are right? That they are right within the confines of a justice system embedded in misogynist ideas? In this system of thought, only women who appear weak or hysterical-in-tears inspire caretaking? Is that how it goes? The rest of us who appear in some manner as 'strong', or who respond not with tears but clarity in response to injustice, well, apparently, we can fend for ourselves? Is that the idea?
Fabiola spoke firmly.
Yeah, that's the idea.
"I hate this idea and all that goes with it!" I exclaimed in frustration.

Fabiola joined me.

Yes, I do too!

She elaborated:

If you go into a meeting and strongly advocate for yourself and try to hold the system accountable, you have to consider that it's going to backfire. That they'll put you into the 'difficult woman' category instead and will now definitely not have your back.

Fabiola clearly did not play the roles of a failed, broken and assaulted self convincingly enough. Setting the counsel to play a docile and meek victim to one side, Fabiola instead invented her own counsel: she imagined both a "little girl" whom she had been, and the "woman" she would be after the January court date, insisting that her conversations take place between these two "authorities" in her life, whom she now recognized as such.

"I have been feeling the presence of my little girl self with me as of late. It feels like she wants to tell me something." Listen to the counsel of what Fabiola called the "little girl":

she says:

you carried me
all these years
in the hollow of your heart
so you listen to me now:
cry to me
before the events make their home in your body
and store themselves there
put on a song for me
and let the shell fall apart, honey
you'll see
I'll emerge from the shell
with faith:
fear shall not rule you
and you will see the barren landscape
break into a hundred wild and flowery paths one more intriguing
than the next
and you will be okay.
your life is not on trial
and by the power invested in me
I order your soul
to be free to roam.

In the same conversation, Fabiola also invoked and imagined the woman whom she was becoming, and whom she wanted to keep close to her in her moments of fear and doubt. She came up with this image in response to my question:

> If you do not want to hold yourself accountable to the opinion of your friends, or the representatives to the legal system, like the police or the prosecutor, whom do you choose instead?

Fabiola took a breath, and uttered:

> I am accountable to the other victims. That's who I am doing this for.

I choked up with tears in response, which kept me silent.
She elaborated and said beneath her tears:

> And you know I have this vision of the woman I will be after the court date is all over. I want to make her proud. All the steps I take now are to make the woman I will be proud of how I went about this.
> This woman, this January woman, is she with you now?
> Yes, I notice her in a certain kind of gravitas that is with me, even now in the way that I walk.
> What have you and your efforts been promising her?
> That I will move towards...something beautiful. Even as some people contribute to ugliness. I want to shield myself in beauty.

I notice her in the weight of my step
in the gravitas that comes from these significant steps
I am taking now

I know the route I have to step
even though I am afraid
of backfirings and the lostness they may cause:

I want to tell my story for her
I want to

put up lights
and campaign for a camera
in this arena
of my appearance.
but it is a delicate balance between joy and depression

all I know is
I need to be moving towards something beautiful
even as
some people contribute to ugliness
I want to shine so bright in it
and seek the beauty
that is my shield

in the end
they said their feeble "fair enough"
and "I shouldn't have said that"
because I held them accountable.

what they don't know is
that I
account to
the woman I will be
and the beauty that is possible for her
after this
particular
winter war.

Chapter 7: Nobody's Ex

As our final reflection, Fabiola and I offer a writ and instruction to therapists assisting those who have suffered mistreatment by "exes" of all kinds, as well as to all of us humans whose imaginations have ever been forcibly captured in the "petty arenas" of others' malice. Listen closely:

Nobody's Ex

Be nobody's ex
looked at
in your brave front
or stared at
in some talk about the brokenness of the past

be an ex-ile
part of the festivities
if you choose
but capable
of lifting your eyes above
and beyond to the future
hoped-for
and willed-toward
by every ordinary step

be nobody's ex
or girlfriend-to-be

be Fabiola
in an upside-down world
of upended social conventions
neither damsel in distress nor abuser
neither master nor servant
neither princess nor broken

be nobody's ex
but qualified

to a free voice and eyes
above and beyond
a past
a present
and a future
as sparkly and magical
as all carnival.

As my closing words, I would like to add a poem by Florence Brooks Whitehouse (2017) that stands as a tribute to Fabiola's achievements in our conversations and in her life: to claim the "clean, clear right to hold her life her own:"

I have no quarrel with you

I have no quarrel with you; but I stand
For the clear right to hold my life my own;
The clean, clear right. To mould it as I will,
Not as you will, with or apart from you;
To make it a thing of brain and blood,
Of tangible substance and of turbulent thought.
No thin gray shadow of the life of man.
Your love, perchance, may set a crown upon it;
But I may crown myself in other ways.
As you have done who are one flesh with me.
I have no quarrel with you – but henceforth,
This you must know; the world is mine, as yours,
The pulsing strength and passion and heart of it;
The work I set my hand to, women's work,
Because I set my hand to it.

Note

1 For more information about the practice of poetry as therapeutic documentation see Behan (2013), Paljakka (2018), Linnell (2004), and Speedy (2008).

References

Behan, P. C. (2013). Rescued speech poems: Co-authoring poetry in narrative therapy. Retrieved: www.narrativeapproaches.com

Brooks Whitehouse, F. (2017). I have no quarrel with you. Published in A. Chagnot, & E.Ikkanda (Eds). *How lovely the ruins: Inspirational poems and words for difficult times.* New York: Penguin Random House (p. 135).

Linnell, S. (2004). Towards a po-ethics of therapeutic practice: Expending the relationship of ethics and aesthetics in narrative therapies through a consideration of the late work of Michel Foucault. *International Journal of Narrative Therapy and Community Work, 4*, 42–54.

Paljakka, S. (2018). A house of good words: A Prologue to the practice of writing poems as therapeutic documents. *Journal of Narrative Family Therapy,* 49–71.

Speedy, J. (2008). *Narrative inquiry and psychotherapy.* Basingstoke: Palgrave Macmillan.

CHAPTER 5

BLOSSOMING IN THE STORM

Sasha McAllum Pilkington

In the Hospice Inpatient Unit

I knocked on the door of 川 Chuan's[1] room and waited. When I heard a faint murmur in response, I stepped inside. Chuan lay in a large reclining chair by the window. Tufts of black hair framed her face, and her smooth golden skin hid the trails of illness. Her eyes stared at the ceiling. I moved closer. "Ni hao Chuan." Only Chuan's eyes moved as she looked at me.

"Hello Sasha." Her voice had lost its musical lightness. I sat down on the edge of the bed hoping my presence might offer some comfort. Chuan reached out and grasped my hand. It was the first time we had touched in the two years we had known each other.

I first met Chuan when she requested counseling following an operation. Cancer had caused the bones in her arm to crumble, and a pin had been put in to hold her bones together. I visited Chuan at home as is usual in my role as a community counselor working in palliative care. From our first meeting I respected Chuan's way of living and integrity. Chuan was married to 山 Shan and they had a son 康 Kang who was 12-years-old. They had migrated to New Zealand from China. Mandarin was their first language, but Chuan kindly accommodated me by speaking English. There were few counselors who spoke Mandarin in

DOI: 10.4324/9781003226543-7

Auckland and none in palliative care. When we first met, I got to know Chuan through her love for Shan and Kang and her compassion. She was a preschool teacher and highly respected in the community.

Sometime later, we decided to write this story together. Chuan hoped other people might learn from her experience.

Six Months Earlier: Opening Doors of Possibility

I could hear voices speaking Mandarin as I climbed the outside stairs to the second level of the house. When I reached the deck at the top of the stairs, I looked down at the mangroves in the estuary below. I imagined it could be a soothing view for someone forced to remain at home. The voices stopped as the TV was turned off.

> Ni hao Chuan!
> "Ni hao Sasha!" Chuan laughed.

From her position on the sofa Chuan groped for a chair for me before falling back from the effort. The large black chair remained in its original place. She smiled, more focused on welcoming me than her own exhaustion. I completed the task and moved the chair around to face Chuan conscious of my relative strength and agility even though I was a decade older than her. I didn't want to bring forward loss for her by emphasizing my capability.

I sat on the chair and returned Chuan's smile. "It's so good to see you Chuan. How did the visit with your family go?"

> "It was great! I was in heaven!" Chuan almost sang.
> You were in heaven?!

Chuan's reply tumbled out as if she could barely contain herself.

> My sister-in-law is very good at massaging ... and my sister. My brother and sister did all the cooking.

I imagined the feel of a good massage and lovingly cooked food.

> Did they come and look after you?

A huge smile engulfed Chuan's face.

> Yes!

I could almost smell the pork buns Chuan loved.

> Was it the cooking and massage that had you in heaven or were there other things as well that were great about their stay?

Chuan laughed as she spoke.

> They just like chatting with me and ask me all the time 'How do you feel?' and "What do you want to eat?" Just feel so good.

I was delighted for her.

> Did you feel loved?

Chuan laughed again.

> Very much!

Chuan shared with me some stories of the time with her family. I encouraged her with questions, aware that such experiences of connection could become increasingly important as she contemplated her approaching death. After a while the conversation turned.

> How do you think your family found staying here and seeing you?

Chuan stopped smiling and the pace of our conversation suddenly slowed. She leaned back in the large leather sofa.

> They worried about me at first but then I get better and it reassuring for them. I felt very bad the week before. My blood cells very low and I had two blood transfusions. My energy level so down and feel depression.

I murmured an acknowledgement and waited to see if she wished to continue. There are usually few occasions when a person can speak freely of the difficult aspects of their experience (see Willing, 2011).
Chuan continued.

> They said when the blood quality is so low people do have depression...it was very bad last week.
>
> What a lot you are forced to manage....

I paused while Chuan nodded her head.

> Would you mind explaining what the depression was like for you?

Chuan bowed her head. Her thick black hair fell across her face, but she didn't tuck it back.

> I just cried and cried. I couldn't stop. Feel despair.

I reflected on the overwhelming feeling of fatigue, so different from tiredness.

> Did the fatigue from the low blood cells take you to a point of despair?

Chuan looked up.

> Yeah. When I went for chemo my red blood cells so low, they did a blood transfusion instead. My family came next day but I need time to recover. My heart was so...it didn't belong to me anymore! I feel exhausted and terrible. I feel like I probably couldn't survive anymore!

Chuan's voice rose in what I imagined was disbelief.
"Oh," I acknowledged, solemn as I responded to the significance of such a declaration. Chuan had withstood so much.
Chuan held her chest as she confided:

> Inside it is all blocked here. The chemotherapy you know.

Chuan's hands remained over her heart (see Chen, Miakowski, Dodd & Pantilat, 2008).

> You said you felt like your heart didn't belong to you anymore....?

Chuan was eager to talk and anticipated my question.

> Feel nervous and angry. I feel worried about everything...is too much and not settle down. Then one of my friends, she's a Buddhist, took me to the Chinese temple. I went to a...what you call...a monk, and he prayed and talk to me. Then my heart settle down.

Chuan sat back on the sofa and her arms fell down to her sides.

I framed my response to draw to Chuan's attention her efforts to influence her life. A sense of agency can help people stave off despair at the end of life (see McClain, Rosenfeld & Breitbart, 2003).

> Would you mind telling me a little more about what you did at the temple that allowed you to settle your heart?
>
> ...Told him I need help. My heart feel horrible and beating...and then he prayed something and play meditation music. It calmed me. Listen, it very beautiful.

Chuan reached over to the table beside her. The soothing sound of a flutist began playing what I guessed was Eastern music.

I reflected on Chuan's ability to make such a request for help.

> You've spoken about talking with the monk and the music. How have you used what the monk shared with you?
>
> The music is for meditation and I doing it every day. It calm me down. It is support for the spirit. After seeing the monk, I listen to the music, and meditate and pray. I can feel my heart is going back to the right position.

Chimes sounded as the music continued in the background seeming to underline her words.

We talked about the difference Chuan's new daily routine was making for her. As we talked, I listened for how Chuan was responding especially if they were in ways that she valued. I then asked her more about the visit.

> Can you tell me a little bit more of what it was like at the temple?

Chuan seemed to glow.

> It's like a family and they are so warm. Everybody is caring for each other's sickness. The monk was very kind and support me. I feel like a reassure.... I've got someone to help me and I feel more hopeful.

Hope can mean many things to people especially when someone has an incurable life-threatening illness. I wondered what it was to Chuan.

> Can you help me understand a little more about this hopefulness and what it means to you?

Wonder entered Chuan's voice.

> "I can feel it when I pray and chant.... I feel like the Buddha is touching me. I feel light from inside my body," Chuan mimed the light flowing from the top of her head down her body, "...and I calm down. I imagine that and just feel better."

I felt honored that she could share such an intimate spiritual experience.

> "What is it like when you feel the light going down your body?" I asked.

I didn't know what would be significant for Chuan.
Chuan answered readily.

> It feel warm and good.
>> How does it affect your ability to calm yourself?

I named "calming" as an ability and something Chuan was doing. She might want to develop it for the future.
Chuan smiled.

> I feel very calm and even though the pain is still there... feel more positive about it.
> "What do you make of that?" I asked.

Chuan spoke quickly as if reciting a well-known fact or the words of someone else.

> It feels like I can accept everything and less complain. I accept it as part of my life experience and Buddha will support me. It's like everybody will have their own problem not just me get sick. It's just part of life.
> "When the cancer and symptoms feel part of life, what difference does that make *to you*?" I asked.
> It's like it's going to be part of my experience. People have different life experience. It's just the way it is but the Buddha will direct and help me to go through that suffering. Not alone.

Chuan smiled as she spoke, cueing me that the sense of companionship might be helpful to her. What she had voiced was different from her previous understandings and so I pursued it.

> When you have a sense of not being alone, how does that change the way you experience suffering?

Chuan's voice softened.

> Feel like company and caring from other people. The feeling of loneliness get better. When I pray, I can imagine the Buddha is touching me. Feel the light.

I noticed Chuan described herself as imagining.

> You said when you pray you can imagine the Buddha is touching you and you feel the light. What kind of imagining do you do, to feel the Buddha's touch?

I was seeking to highlight Chuan's knowledge in generating such an experience.

> I imagine the lightness will go down and warm my body and the water will wash it clean.

Chuan brushed her hands down her body.

> That feeling very good.
> "Mmm," I murmured in wonder.

I was unfamiliar with what Chuan had just shared. We sat in silence for a moment with the sun streaming in.
Chuan continued.

> I was thinking about spiritual help for a long time. You remember I tried a Christian church too? I tried so many things. I think this is the right choice for me because the Buddha is from the tradition of Eastern culture.
> "What are you prioritizing that's important to you when you draw on knowledge from Eastern traditions?" I asked.

Chuan seemed to meditate on the question.

> It is a philosophy for the people. It is part of life...it depends, I listen to many ideas.

I reflected on her skill in doing such listening in a country where she wasn't born.

> How do you go about deciding which ideas you will draw on?

Chuan pointed to the Chinese herbs on the table and a steamer that her family had brought from China.

> I learn about anything that might help. I'm keep practicing qi gong and steaming. I'll carry on the chemotherapy. All trying to help. I think it's positive and it make your body accept and not fighting.

I noted her comment of not fighting.

> Is your body 'accepting' rather than 'fighting' more useful to you?
> Yeah.

Chuan looked at me as if waiting for more.

> Could you help me understand a little more of what you mean when you speak of your body accepting?
> "Acceptance" could carry so many meanings in the context of illness and dying.
> Even the cancer is part of my body. I meditate and try to get the cancer cell to be neutral not active, make them sleepy...harmonious.
> Harmonious!

I repeated the word, captivated by the idea.

> "Harmony of the body," Chuan enthused.

She was looking as if she was delighted by my interest (see Chen, Miakowski, Dodd & Pantilat, 2008).

> You've said the cancer cells are you...and you're looking to calm them, to put them to sleep, to be harmonious. How does this harmonious state influence your wellbeing?

Chuan's face softened, and a small smile played around the edges of her mouth.

> It's like...we can survive together.
>> Survive together.
>
> "Wow" I thought to myself. It was so different from Western ideas of how people should live with cancer.

Chuan suddenly grinned.

> You now know the new philosophy of the Chinese doctor!

I smiled back warmly. Chuan began sharing with me examples that illustrated what she wanted to convey.

> If someone was watching you day by day, what would they notice about you that would tell them that you were surviving together with the cancer?

Chuan sat back, looking thoughtful. She answered slowly as she contemplated.

> They probably notice my tempers been better. More happy, and my family atmosphere is better. Maybe my temper and the tension influenced everyone and made us argue. This week we are all harmonious. We're trying to talk to each other in a gentle voice. We're a lot happier.

Chuan laughed.

> Have you spread the harmony from this 'surviving together' relationship you have with the cancer... to the family?

I was wishing Shan could join the conversation. He was now the sole income earner and busy at work.
Surprise was in Chuan's tone as she answered.

> Yeah! ...I'm trying to change my son's behavior so I have to change myself first. I'm trying to talk with him in a gentle voice and be more tolerant of his behavior. Even if he get angry, I won't argue with him. I will let him calm down first and talk about it later. That's my new technology!

Chuan finished with a conspiratorial laugh one mother to another. I joined in, appreciative of her wisdom.

I continued to work at strengthening the newly revealed links.

> As you've learnt these things, what difference has it made to your experience of the cancer and the way you live with it?

Chuan leaned forward on the sofa.

> I'm brave now. Still experience lots of pain and bad feeling but I am growing with cancer. I learned a lot from my experience. I have spent the most precious time with my son instead of working. The money's not always important you know. I listen to my body and respect it. It's for my family too. You're not just yourself! My courage is back, and I can handle it more with the help of my husband and friends. I can accept it more calmly.

I appreciated Chuan's ability to see herself as connected to others. Cancer doesn't just happen to one person. I also noted the way she cherished time with her son Kang. People often feel pressured to find the good in hard situations, but this had come wholly from Chuan with acknowledgment of the hard times. I considered asking her about her courage but instead took another direction.

> What is it that you can accept more calmly?
> Accept the fact I have cancer and still life threatening...but more calmly.

This was the first conversation where I had heard Chuan touch on her approaching death without panic or fear.

Chuan and I continued to talk. I discovered how she had inspired her friends. I learnt of what she gave to her family by the way she received their gifts. I wondered what might sustain her as she was forced to contemplate the end of her life.

Towards the end of our time together I asked:

> How has this conversation gone for you today? Have we talked about what you hoped, or have I taken us a bit off track?

I wanted the conversation to be what Chuan had hoped for. Chuan assured me the conversation had been as she had wished.

It was late and I needed to get back to the hospice. As I walked out through the sliding door, I turned to say a final goodbye. Chuan's eyes were wide open.

> Sasha, I didn't know I was like that before....I didn't know I was strong...I didn't know I knew that! Thank you.

I left, wishing I could have asked her more.

Stories Through the Generations

> My memory getting bad these days. It's side effect from my new chemo.

Chuan was updating me when we met a month later.

We were sitting in her living room with the sun shining in through the large windows that overlooked the hillside. It was just after Chinese New Year. Special sweet treats were on the table, and I caught sight of a red envelope that was likely Kang's. I murmured an acknowledgment. There were many challenges, not just those the illness posed. The cancer that was part of Chuan's body was progressing and, as first line treatments failed, she had been prescribed new chemotherapy with significant side effects.

> How does that impact on your day to day living?

I looked at the cap Chuan now wore. As she had predicted, her hair had fallen out.

> I remember good things, the bad things easy to forget. I have to write down all my appointments. Memory's getting worse. That's sad, aye.

Chuan laughed. I remained solemn. I was curious about the disparity in what she remembered.

> How do you go about remembering the good things that you want to remember?

Chuan giggled.

> Still can remember...it's quite funny. It's like the good things give me deep impressions.

I was drawn to Chuan's description. I often noticed how her constructions of English led me to richer understandings of what she wanted to convey.

Chuan chuckled, her eyes sparkling:

Like when my son was a baby time, I can remember all the funny things. The funny things he did make me laugh.
   Would you mind sharing a story of a fun time you had with Kang?

Chuan and I had previously agreed to preserve any stories she wanted to share with Kang. They were to make up part of an ethical will that she would leave him. Chuan talked about Kang when he was a baby. I asked her questions, so the stories became fuller versions than those she usually told. Chuan described how Kang liked to imitate accents, especially a New Zealander trying to speak Mandarin, when the language was unfamiliar to them. We were both soon laughing.
   I asked mischievously:

How did he do? What was the accent like?.

I was delighted Chuan felt comfortable to share a joke about the group I belonged to.
   Chuan laughed as she replied:

It's so funny. You probably think it's good 'cos you don't know the way we speak Chinese, but we know what the proper accent should be! Kiwi[2] people can't make certain sound you know. Kang making the accent just sounds so funny! Make me laugh.
   Well, I'll make sure I learn from you and not Kang!

I joked, following Chuan's lead that this was a light-hearted moment. She laughed again. I reflected on how much fun we had together in amongst conversations of loss and suffering. Sometimes I thought our conversations reflected both the savoring of life as well as the harshness.

Who else in the family has a good sense of humor?
   "My husband, his side of the family...Probably me too... I like funny things. Maybe I got it from my father," Chuan chortled.
   Have you got a story about your father's humor that you could share?

Chuan became serious as she explained:

> He is actually like a two-sided. When he is happy, he is so happy. He could be fine and have a sense of humor. But sometime, you know he is black with his bad memories, the story of his early age. And he will be just so sad, especially when it is Chinese New Year. He remembers his Mom and Dad.
>
> Did he mourn his Mom and Dad at Chinese New Year?

I often asked questions that clarified and summarized to support our communication. I wanted to do all I could, especially given that Chuan was using valuable energy and concentration by speaking English to accommodate me.

Chuan nodded as she pondered her Dad's sorrow.

> Yeah, sad.

As respectfully as I could I asked:

> How did he go about that mourning? What did he do that told you he was feeling sad?
>
> You can see he's sad...at that time...very cries. Sometime, he will just tell us a story about when he was young and when he had hard time starving. His mom was sick in bed and he got no food. He remember that and tell us about it.

I tried to absorb what she was telling me.

> Would you mind explaining a little more about that?...What was his mom sick from?
>
> Sick from poverty. He got no food, and the people all get very weak and easy to catch all the bugs you know.

Silently, tears gathered in the corners of Chuan's eyes.

Death from starvation and poverty was suddenly personal. I tried to imagine what it was like for Chuan's Dad as I stuttered:

> From poverty and starvation...she was sick...and he was hungry?

Chuan seemed to respond to my measured congruence.

> Yeah...'cos that was the time when Japan invaded China and lots of people, they've got no home and no food. We live in the Northeast parts of China and then, when the war start, there is nowhere to go. They have to go to the South...and everywhere people poor. No food and no shelter and I think his mom died from that.

Again, intentionally letting some of my reaction show I asked:

> His mom died from starvation and poverty?

I wanted to respond, showing my recognition of the importance of Chuan's story, while still centering her.
Tears rolled down Chuan's face.

> Yeah... and sickness. It's easy to get sick when you're very weak and they don't have money to pay for the doctor. No way!
> "No," I acknowledged.

Chuan lowered her voice and I leant forward to hear her not wanting to miss a word.

> Even for the food.... Starving you know.

More tears escaped her eyes.
"And his father?" I almost whispered.

> His father...when Japan was in the North part of China they need people, labor for the coal mine. My father's father, my grandpa, was cheated by one of the people from the mine. The man said, 'You can get good money. You go work there.' My Dad's father and grandpa went together with that man to the mine, and they never came back. They died. Nobody know. Just buried in the mine I think.

We were both fully focused on the story, giving Chuan's family our respect.

> Oh, how terrible!

> Yes, this terrible. So many people killed. They just trick, cheap labor to work for them. They never get good pay, and they could not escape from there. They die.

I tried to imagine what such a history was like for her family. I considered the impact such stories might have on the way Chuan made meaning of her life as she faced the challenges of living with cancer.

> What sort of effect has that background had...on the family, and what you've learnt...and come to value and appreciate?

Chuan remained silent. I realized my question was unclear and decided to break it down into smaller inquiries. While we had often talked about how to manage me not being able to speak Mandarin, Chuan was hesitant when I was unclear and often tried to work out my meaning. I therefore remained alert for questions that could be confusing.

> I'm sorry. That was a jumble of ideas. Would you mind if I reworded the question?

Chuan indicated I should go ahead, her eyes on me.

> How has that sorrow affected the family, do you think, going down the generations?

She responded immediately.

> It's like we should never forget... that history. And as a nation we should work hard and get a better life. It's better not to have that happen again. We have education at school...we need to work hard and be independent...economically. It's like a nation's things pass onto generation after generation. Don't forget that history.
>
> What is it about the history that's important for *you* not to forget?

As Chuan spoke I listened for her values.

> I would like my son to grow up be a good people and don't never do bad things to other people and other nation. I want him to be a kind person.

133

That was terrible animal behavior before. I want that never to happen to him.

Is kindness something that is important to you?

Chuan sat up straight as she stated:

That's what I think yeah. Be a human being. Be a good people you know. You can't do bad thing to other nation or other people. That's just horrible. I would like him to grow up kind. Also, I want him to be a useful person, an independent person. Have a happy life.

I repeated, to check that I had understood her:

Kind, a useful person, an independent person, and have a happy life.

Chuan nodded relaxing her posture.

Like he can have his own skill and survive. I want him to grow up like that.

Implicit in our conversation was the knowledge Chuan wouldn't see Kang grow up, giving added weight to her declaration.

We've spoken in the past of your compassion…I asked you a lot about starting as a preschool teacher…does some of that compassion have its roots in your family history and also in what you want to pass on to your son?

Not only did I want to bring forward for Chuan her legacy, but it's possible history and continuity as she made sense of her life and approaching death.

I think so. Being my dad grown up like that, want us to be kind people.
How do you understand your Dad wanting you to be kind rather than say angry, even though he'd seen his mother die of illness from starvation and his father killed without the family being told what happened?

Speaking on her father's behalf Chuan stated:

He had been treated very badly by some people.

I replied firmly.

> Yes.

My strong affirmative seemed to encourage Chuan to move further into the story. Tears flowed down her face. Her tone became plaintive.

> But he think it not fair...and people shouldn't do that to other people.
>> "Was he a principled person?" I suggested, offering her words to consider.

Chuan lent forward as she wept, "Yes."

> ...Somebody who believed in justice?

Chuan nodded, seeming unable to speak.

We sat in silence. I thought about what a remarkable man Chuan's father was. I wondered if he considered himself in such a way.

> Would you say he has passed on that value of justice and...doing the right thing, to you?

Chuan found her voice.

> I can remember when we were young there were still some people who live in very bad condition and very poor. They begging for food. When we have some, we always give them some. Share you know...

"Oh," I uttered, as I reflected on their generosity.

> My Dad he knew what it was like to starve. He had that experience and he, when he can, always help other people. Yeah...if you can, always help.

Chuan clutched her chest her eyes wet with emotion. I stuttered, moved with admiration:

> Is that something you're proud of in your family? That you've turned the cruelty of war....such a terrible experience...into a desire to...be kind?

I wanted to draw Chuan's attention to the ways the family had responded to hardship. Such stories could create landscapes of agency for her to draw on as loss wove itself into her day to day life.

> I'm so proud of my father. He was a good person even though he experienced that. He learnt from the good side of life, not the bad side. Always been very kind...a good person.

Chuan choked as her tears flowed.
I was moved by her love and respect for her father.

> Chuan, does it make any difference to you to be connected to your father, to his integrity and kindness as you live with this cancer?

Chuan furrowed her brow thinking.

> I think of my daddy's life and know I am so lucky even though I have cancer. I got lots of people to help and new medicines. I have hope and very grateful. My daddy's life far worse than me but still he survived and had a life and a family. I think my father is very powerful in that part. He grew out of it and struggled but still survived. I'm so proud of him.

I noticed Chuan's irrepressible ability to see luck in her life, to feel grateful. I decided to return to it later and learn more. I thought of her father's story and the story tracing the integrity of her mother's family that I had heard previously.

> What is it like to be part of a family who even when things are terrible turn to goodness rather than anger or hatred?

Chuan reflected and then replied firmly.

> It's very powerful and helpful.

I asked Chuan about how such knowledge was helpful to her. I remembered Chuan's dad had died only a year ago. We spent the next half an hour talking about how the legacy of Chuan's dad showed up in her life. I brought her mom into the conversation and learnt that Chuan had courage like her mom. I then turned the conversation to Kang. Like many parents of young children, leaving Kang was the most painful thought for Chuan to contemplate. We were gathering stories for a therapeutic document for Kang and now I sought to include him in it.

> How do you think Kang is learning about kindness and justice from you?

Chuan immediately answered.

> It's from how I love him. We give each other a cuddle when he come back home. He learn how to love people. He learns from daily experience. I think he is observant, and he learns every day about love.

Chuan rested her head on her hand.

> What does he do that tells you he is learning about love?

Chuan smiled and turned to face me, her eyes crinkling and her voice soft.

> He gives me lots of cuddles and when I feel ill, he will ask me, 'How do you feel, Mom? Are you okay?,' 'Momma, I'll give you a kiss and you'll feel better.' It's those sweet things. Make me happy…feel loved.

I nodded warmly, appreciating Kang.

> Is there anything else that springs to mind that shows Kang's knowledge of loving?

I was keen to bring forward what Kang was giving to his mom. The gifts of young people can easily be overlooked.
Chuan shared with me many ways that Kang was helping her.

> "My son make me laugh. My friend bought me a bag…my son told me, "Mom, I think this bag is for old woman. Not for you, you are young and pretty."

137

Chuan laughed heartily.

> "Oh!" I exclaimed in delight.
> What was it like to be told by your son you are young and pretty?!
> I was laughing.... He was so serious. He try to persuade me. No, no, Mom you still young and pretty.
> And in that moment did you get a look of yourself through his eyes and feel young and pretty?
> I just laughed.

The joy of her laughter seemed cocooned in love.

> What did your husband think?
> He was laughing too!

I smiled.

> What's it like to know that Kang thinks you are young and pretty?
> I think he probably does think I'm young and pretty! Very happy and feel quite proud!

Chuan lent back on the sofa with a big grin on her face.

> What do you feel proud of?

Chuan's face glowed.

> Proud of...how do you say...proud of the way he is and the way he look at me.

I imagined Kang with his mom.

> What difference does it make to be looked at as young and pretty and be loved by your son as you live with this cancer?

Chuan considered.

> I feel I have more reason to look after myself...it's for my son. I have to treat myself good and if I can, live longer...give me courage as well.

I wonder what it will be like for him when he is older to know that he made you feel happy, gave you purpose in looking after yourself, and inspired your courage?

"I will tell him if I can. I will tell him how important it is for me to hear his word and know about it and give me hope."

Chuan seemed to reflect and laughed again. I responded to her amusement.

"I wonder what ideas he has about the kind of handbag you should have?"

Later I gathered my bags and got ready to leave. As I stood up, Chuan again said:

"I didn't know that about myself, Sasha. I didn't know that about my family."

There could have been pride in her voice.

Second by Second

Upon sitting down, I asked:

> Where do you think would be a good place to start?

I had been away, and a month had passed since we last met. Chuan sat on the sofa. Wisps of barely visible hair covered her head, and I could see the effects of steroids lingering in her cheeks.

> I don't know. I've just kind of lost my voice 'cos I got a cough recently. The doctor say it may be side effect of my new chemo. Just started it. Apologise. On off the cough. It quite annoying sometime.

I immediately considered the possible impact of our conversation on Chuan.

> How is talking going to be for you then?
> It's okay, but not too much maybe.

Chuan cleared her throat.
I lowered my voice aware of my concern for her.

> Not too much.... How will you know when you're getting towards the end of what you can comfortably do?

Chuan explained screwing up her face:

> Cough...cough. And I have to stop for a little while.
> Okay. Would that be a sign that we should stop our conversation and I go, or how would you envisage it?

Chuan's face relaxed.

> We can see how it goes.
> Okay, I don't want to over tax your voice, alright?

I replied, smiling to remind her that I was on her team, and she was who mattered. I suspected it might be hard for her to tell me she wanted to stop.

Chuan's face seemed to light up.

> It's alright.

I smiled again and in an easy tone tried to create more space for her to tell me how she was.

> ...So, I'm counting on you letting me know early.

I resolved to watch out for any signs Chuan might be tiring or her voice being taxed.

Chuan nodded smiling back at me.

> Yeah, I will. I am very happy to meet you all time. Give me lots of help. Like I understand a lot of myself when I feel bad and allow myself to cry. From all the pain, all the suffering you know. Not bad thing. I used to think I am so weak and not a good strong person. I would criticise myself when I cry, but you gave me the chance to understand there's a good side actually.

I hadn't expected what Chuan had just shared. I cast my mind back to conversations where we had talked about crying. All I could remember was asking Chuan about what her tears were expressing from time to time.

> Would you mind sharing a little more about that?
>
> Feel quite negative about when I feel sad...I feel so weak not strong enough. When I cry I just kind of blame myself. But you helped me to understand it's okay to be sad and it's not negative things. Actually, give me lots of help about that.

I hadn't been aware that Chuan was developing some new beliefs about expressing her sadness. I wondered if the action of inquiring into her distress and the process of respecting and companioning her tears could be powerful without actually talking much about it head on. I reflected that even passing tissues can inadvertently give a message of "stop crying."

Would it be okay if I asked you a few questions about that?

Chuan nodded.

Yeah sure.
What different understandings do you hold about expressing sadness now, that you didn't have previously?
In my education, in my background, my culture not good to cry…when I cry, I always criticised.

Tears spilled onto Chuan's cheeks.

Told 'Stop crying, you silly girl,' that sort of things.
"How do you think people developed those ideas?" I inquired.

Chuan looked out the window briefly before returning to face me.

I think it was from their life. Struggle to survive. The society was very cruel for them. There was a root from that, I think. They have to be strong and not show emotion. Not allowed to cry and show weakness. I thought that too, but then think about what we talk about…and about time with operation. I didn't want to think about it before. Very terrible…make me so scared…hard time.

Chuan clasped her shoulder. I remembered how her bone had been pinned after the cancer had caused it to break. Her recovery had been long and difficult. Tears forged their way down Chuan's face in spite of her attempts to wipe them away.
Tentatively I checked:

Would you like to talk about what happened in that hard time?

Chuan replied immediately. Small sobs escaped her as she spoke.

It was the night…I was in so much pain from the operation…. The pain was terrible. They numb you but the drugs already gone. I did take some oral pain killer but just not strong enough. The pain was still there…. It was horrible.

Chuan began to cry unreservedly.

> So terrible. I didn't know how I would get through the night.

My voice was low.

> How awful. What did you do? How did you manage to get through that night with such terrible pain?

Still weeping she explained:

> I couldn't do anything. So bad....I counted second by second by second for that night.

I tried to imagine such an experience. I noted that Chuan felt she hadn't done anything and reflected that feeling powerless was usually unhelpful and especially when approaching death. I started to search for how Chuan responded reminding myself that counting was doing something,

> What did counting, second by second, do?
> > It just tell me time passing. Only way I could know...so bad.
>
> Chuan wrapped her arms around herself and drew her knees up to her chin.
>
> Could you help me understand what was important about knowing that the time was passing?
> > Only way to survive...knowing it must end sometime. Thought if I get through one second then I move onto the next second. All I could do.
>
> Can I check that I've understood you properly? To survive the agonizing pain, you kept hold of the knowledge that it might end sometime...and got through the night by counting each second?
> > Yeah, I did that.

Chuan looked up at me unfolding her body from its semi-cocooned position.

> What did you draw on that allowed you to do that?
> > Need my courage. I need it all, so terrible the pain.

I reflected on our recent explorations of Chuan's courage, and her comment that she had not known she had courage before. I wondered if re-connecting her to such courage had helped to make this conversation possible.

Chuan's eyebrows drew together as she explained further:

> I had to keep calling the nurses. I thought maybe if they change my position for me, it might help but just not work. But I feel sorry for them so busy.

I was struck by her ability to feel for another person at such a moment.

> Did you feel sorry for the nurses even though you were in terrible pain?!

Chuan leant forward, sounding indignant.

> Other patients yelling at them. They were trying their best but some people very rude.
>
> When you called the nurses, do you think they noticed that you were feeling for them?
>
> They say I'm sweet and they try to help me. They say I'm not like the other people who were shouting at them. One nurse tried many time to fix my pillows, and make me comfortable. They tell me to call them and say they will come straight away.

I wasn't surprised to hear this. Chuan's kindness and humility stood out to me.

> What do you think they noticed about you that led them to think you were sweet and someone they wanted to reassure they would help immediately?
>
> They know I have pain and don't want to bother them. They can tell that I feel for them. I use soft voice and polite. They trying their best. Doing everything they can for all the people. They very good to me actually. Even if they can't help they still trying ....feel support.

I reflected on how much I enjoyed time with Chuan.

> What do you make of your ability to form this kind of relationship with the nurses?

Chuan considered and then in a soft tone replied:

> I think I might be like my Dad. We always think of other people....

She paused a moment, then sat up as if gathering herself and stated:

> ...And courage maybe like my mom...she is brave.

Chuan and I went on to research other stories that showed her capacity to respond compassionately even in hard times. We linked these to the legacy of her family. It wasn't long before I discovered that her family and friends were drawing inspiration from her.

As we talked, I checked in with her regularly as to how she was managing the conversation. Each time Chuan firmly assured me she wanted to talk. Nevertheless, I was careful to leave on time. Fatigue can catch up on a person.

Flowering in the Storm

Six weeks later Chuan sent me a text requesting that we postpone our meeting. She had been admitted into hospital. At the end of the week, I learnt that Chuan had stopped taking all Western medicines and discharged herself from hospital against medical advice. The reason for her departure was unknown. I wondered what had happened. I knew Chuan would have considered reasons for her decisions. I also thought it likely there were obstacles to Chuan speaking openly about her experience in hospital. She was an immigrant and guided by knowledge that may have been unfamiliar to those looking after her.

The hospice team was worried for Chuan. She was very unwell and suddenly stopping her steroid medication was dangerous, even life threatening. After consulting with my colleagues, I telephoned Chuan and Shan and asked if they would like me to visit them that day. They both responded enthusiastically.

Clouds shrouded the hillside above the estuary as I climbed up the stairs of Chuan and Shan's home. Shan greeted me at the door and led me into the bedroom. Chuan was resting on top of the bed. Her eyes were open, but her focus seemed inward. A sick bowl lay beside the bed.

Chuan turned her attention to me.

> Thank you for coming, Sasha.

Relief layered her tone.

> It's good to see you Chuan. Thank you for seeing me when you're feeling so unwell.

Shan hovered in the doorway. He indicated I should sit down, and I pulled a chair around so Chuan could see me without effort.

Chuan sighed but then with more energy than I anticipated said:

> I am very happy to meet you all time. Give me lots of help. Sasha, I had terrible time in hospital! Thought I was going to go crazy! No sleep for three days. An old person keep our room awake every night. Asked for another room but there is none. Was going crazy!

I tried to imagine having no sleep for three nights when very sick with advanced cancer. I couldn't.

> No sleep for three days! I imagine you're exhausted! No wonder you felt like you were going crazy.
>> Yes, going crazy. No choice, had to leave. Couldn't stay!

Chuan had good reasons for leaving hospital.

> Did you leave to get some much needed rest?

Panic seemed to edge its way into Chuan's voice as she spoke.

> Yes. Feel very terrible. Pain in head and can't remember things. Been falling over for no reason. No one know why. Shan had to carry me up the stairs.
>> You fell over for no reason? ....Did this happen out of the blue?
>
> Just happen. No warning. My legs suddenly not holding me up. Lucky I not hurt.

She moved restlessly on the bed.

> Thank goodness you weren't hurt....Were you scared?

Chuan and I began to go over a little of what had been happening to her. She then raised the topic of her medication.

> I stopped all Western medicine. Just doing acupuncture now....

Tentatively I inquired further.

> Would you mind me asking, what led to your decision?
>> Worried about side effects.... On too many pills....

I reflected on some of the challenges that came with medication. Weighing up possible benefits versus the disadvantages could be a murky task. It wasn't always the straightforward process people expected.
As respectfully as I could I asked:

> Did you have any particular concerns about the steroid?

147

Chuan explained she believed it wasn't helping.

Tentatively I asked:

> Our doctor wanted me to check with you....I imagine it may not have been explained or it could have slipped your mind since you are managing so much... but did you know that stopping the steroid suddenly is dangerous?

Chuan immediately looked concerned and indicated she hadn't known this.

I continued:

> ...If you want to stop it our doctor could help you do so safely. Would you consider talking about it with her?

Usually, I am rigorous in taking a position of not knowing about medical matters. A position of naïve inquirer allows me to be alongside people and hear their concerns from a unique vantage point. I want people to have the space to explore what is right *for them*. However, working in a multi-disciplinary team can be helpful to achieve this. Chuan had been distressed in hospital and understandably unable to hear what the doctors had said about suddenly stopping the powerful steroid she had been prescribed. The hospice team wanted her to have the best chance of making an informed choice and had requested that I raise this safety issue with her inside the comfort of our relationship. Our doctors would then follow up.

I knew Chuan to be a thoughtful person who took care of her wellbeing. Our conversation flowed easily. Shan joined us and together we discussed what they might do next should Chuan continue to experience the unexplained symptoms. A week later, Chuan decided to come into the hospice inpatient unit. However, first she was scheduled to have a scan of her brain in hospital.

Full Circle

I sat on Chuan's bed in the hospice. Chuan held my hand. Her fingers seemed to reach into the familiarity of our relationship for comfort. The results of the scan had arrived. The cancer was throughout Chuan's brain. She was dying. Chuan, Shan and I were reflecting on her life.

> What sort of life would you say you've had, Chuan?
> I've had a good life but now it is my time.
> Can I ask you Chuan...what is a good life to you?
> A good life for me is....I really admire people who, even when they having a hard time, they are showing their beauty to other people like a flower, even though the weather is bad it still blossom. I think that is a good life.

In awe I repeated:

> .... A flower...that shows its beauty...

Chuan smiled slightly:

> Even in very bad weather...in very bad situation...they still blossom. It is so great.

I paused soaking up the image.

> If your family and friends were here, how do you think they might describe *you*?

Chuan considered.

> Maybe my story will give inspiration to someone...

A few days later I sat by Chuan. It was lunchtime and Shan was on the telephone in the next room organizing support for Kang. Chuan lay unmoving in the bed. I listened to the sound of her breathing and offered what companionship I could. I left not long after Shan returned. It was time for my team meeting. Health and safety, cars, staffing, and then it was over. By habit I looked down towards the inpatient unit as I left the meeting room. My head jerked. The candle was lit. Chuan had died.

Notes

1 All names and identifying details have been changed.
2 New Zealander's are often known as "Kiwis."

References

Chen, L., Miakowski, C., Dodd, M. & Pantilat, S. (2008). Concepts within Chinese culture that influence the cancer pain experience. *Cancer Nursing*, 31, 2, 103–108.

McClain, C., Rosenfeld, B. & Breitbart, W. (2003). Effect of spiritual well-being on end-of-life despair in terminally ill cancer patients. *Lancet*, 361, 1603–1607.

Willing, C. (2011). Cancer diagnosis as discursive capture: Phenomenological repercussions of being positioned within dominant constructions of cancer. *Social Science & Medicine*, 73, 897–903.

CHAPTER 6

BATMAN RETURNS
Love and Ethics in Narrative Couples Therapy

Tom Carlson

When I met Megan and Dan in the waiting room for our first couples therapy session, I immediately tentatively concluded that there were considerable grounds for concern.

They were sitting several feet away from each other and staring intently into their phones. After introducing myself to them, we walked back to my office in silence. They walked apart from one another with their heads remaining fixated on their phones. As they took their seats on the couch, I couldn't help but notice that they sat as far apart as possible, turning their backs slightly away from each as if to avoid any eye contact. After introducing myself to them, I asked them if they had any questions about me or what we were about to embark on together.

They spoke in unison but almost inaudibly, both staring at the floor:

I don't think so.

Concerned about them being devoid of any liveliness in their physical and verbal responses, I proceeded asking a question that has become customary in my initial conversations with couples.

Megan and Dan, if you are anything the like other couples who have come to meet me, I am guessing that it was an uncomfortable decision to come here today and as a consequence you might feel ill at ease. And I imagine that whatever trouble your relationship is in, that this is not what you had

> imagined for yourselves when you first decided to begin your relationship together, or that you now find yourselves living in some way contrary to your hopes and dreams for your relationship. Would you mind telling me what it is that is so important to you both that brought you here today to meet someone like me?

I admit that I had anticipated that this question might elicit some kind of a lively response from them, something that might give us something to fight for, but my hopes were quickly dashed. Megan and Dan responded in the same quiet, almost dispirited, tone as they had before, their comments overlapping one another.

> We have just grown so distant over the past year.
>> We hardly talk to each other anymore. We don't even fight. When we go to bed, we just turn over and look at our phones. We no longer even say good night to one another.

When I inquired, Megan and Dan also spoke of a quiet anger and resentment that had been growing between them.

Upon hearing their comments, my concern grew to alarm. In my work with couples over the years, I have found that such a quiet pervasive resentment predicts that the parties to the relationship have become not only resigned to its dissolution but also disengaged from their own lives as well. As a therapist, I would much rather see couples who are fighting, angry, yelling at each other even. At least these are signs of life and liveliness that there is something worth fighting for.

Feeling a sense of urgency to encourage some kind of vitality that might have the effect of turning them toward one another, the following question formed in my mind.

> Megan and Dan, are you okay with treating each other this way, with turning away from each other and the quiet resentment that has come between you?

Dan quickly responded.

> I don't like being angry at her. I don't like resenting her. I feel awful. I call her my better half and my best friend because she really is. It's not okay with me to be angry with her or upset at her. I hate that I feel this way.

Wanting to seize on Dan's dissent at the effects of his actions on Megan, I pressed on.

> Dan, can you help me understand why it is that you say, 'It's not okay for me to be angry at her' and 'I feel awful?'

Tears began to well up in Dan's eyes.

> I want to see her smile again. I think back when we first started dating, which was a long time ago now—almost seven years. I made her laugh a lot. I like making her laugh.

Turning towards Megan for the first time since we were in each other's company, Dan repeated:

> I like making you laugh.

Upon hearing this Megan responded by way of some comic relief.

> Well, you are going to have to come up with some new jokes after all these years. But seriously, I just want to be relaxed again at home. I come home from work and I'm nervous about what his mood is going to be when I get home. Any sign of him having an off day, I instantly go on the defensive. I don't want to be hurt. It sucks to constantly be on edge the entire day. And I definitely don't want to bring a child into this kind of relationship. I know all too well what that is like. I just want to be able to relax and have a good time and be that couple that everyone tells us we are. We have so many friends who say, 'You guys are so perfect together! You guys look great and awesome.' I want to be the couple that we're showing other people. I want to have that great relationship and be models for people.

I admit to being surprised by the way their friends so highly regarded the quality of their relationship in such sharp contrast to their own low regard for it. I couldn't help but notice that there seemed to be an alternative history here. For seven years, their relationship had been a reserve for their good humor. Hoping to somehow bring this alternative history to bear against their current struggles, I asked:

> Is there something about the history of your relationship together that, if I were more familiar with it, might lead me to be a bit surprised at the struggles you are experiencing in your relationship over the past several months?

Megan's eyes lit up and she stated with conviction.

> This might sound lame, but there's a picture from our wedding that my sister said is her favorite picture of us. It shows how much emotion we have. It's our wedding dance. We both have the biggest grins on our face, and you can just see how happy and in love we are. I think if you saw that picture, you would definitely say, 'Wow... why are these two are here today.' I know that was the best day of my life and I was so exhausted at the end of it, but we are that type of people. We wear our emotions 100 per cent. When you see that picture, you see all the emotions of that day.

Here it was. The sign of liveliness that I was hoping for. Sensing that this relationship was far from over, I responded expansively:

> That sounds like a lovely picture. Are there any other emotions that this picture captures about that day and that might give me any clues as to what your relationship has been about?

Megan happily continued.

> He also cried more about the wedding than I did. Dan was so overwhelmed by the emotion we both felt that he couldn't conceal his tears of joy. It's a cute picture of him wiping his tears.
> "I am a big cry baby," Dan said with smile on his face.
> Megan, would you say that is an okay thing, that Dan cried more than you and that he is a bit of a cry baby?
> I love that he has emotions. Love it. Because I have rarely seen my dad cry. The first time that I can remember was at my mom's funeral. That was the first time I saw my dad cry.

Dan jumped in.

I've always been taught it's okay to be in touch with your emotions. I learned that from my dad. He's a very open with his emotions. He even cries more than my mom at sappy movies. That's just him.

Would you say, Dan, that you have received a little different training that we as men normally receive?

Very much so. Yes!

Is that okay with you that you got trained a little differently growing up?

Dan nodded in agreement and Megan added:

I sure hope so. It is one of the things I love most about Dan. If we have boys, I would love our kids to be in touch with their emotions as much as he is. He proposed on Christmas Eve in front of his parents. It was him, me, and his dad crying.

Taken by this image of them all crying joyfully together on Christmas eve, I inquired:

As you imagine the image of you on your wedding day, your wedding dance, your emotions, the smiles, and the joy that it managed to capture and look at that in your mind's eye, does it provide you with some sense of hope that you can get past whatever it is that is besetting your relationship?

Without any hesitation, Megan responded:

I think we've already gotten through a lot in our relationship, and we just don't want to deal with this.

Dan warm-heartedly added:

We've been through so much together. In my mind, there's nothing we can't deal with. Megan's mom passed away four years ago. If we were able to get through that, we should be able to get through anything together.

Has the past year challenged your relationship in ways that have been a bit unfamiliar to you?

Both Megan and Dan agreed that this was indeed so. There was a notable change in the atmosphere in the room. Upon recounting this alternative history, their voices grew more and more vivacious as if their relationship now had some possibility of resurrection. Buoyed by the hope and conviction implicit in this history, I decided to take a risk.

> I am wondering, Megan and Dan, if you two have had a chance to talk with one another about the toll that it has taken on each of you to be living with this distance and quiet resentment, instead of both the love and friendship that had accompanied you during your first several years of your relationship together?

Megan was quick to answer:

> I think that would be really important. I don't think that we have any idea what it is like for the other person. We are always so on guard with each other.

I was not surprised at all by her answer, and asked:

> Would that be of any interest to you both?

Dan hurriedly replied.

> It would be of great interest to me. I would really like to hear what this has been like for Megan.

I smiled at hearing Dan's response, knowing what I was about to ask next.

> I might be asking some questions that are a bit unusual or at least different than what you might think. For example, Dan, rather than asking you what living with these struggles has been like for you personally, I am going to ask you to be a witness to what you think it's been like for Megan to live with the feelings of resentment that you've been having towards her, the distance, the coldness.... Do you have any guesses as to what it's been like for Megan, as a person, to be living with this resentment and coldness over the past several months?

Dan grew quiet as tears began to well up in his eyes.

> I think it's actually been kind of traumatic for her. I've been pretty cold to her at times, and for the longest time I've always been there for her, and I think it's made her feel like I'm not there for her now.
>
> If you were to make your best guess Dan, what do you think it has been like for Megan to not have you there for her?

Tears were now streaming down Dan's face and turning to speak directly to Megan, he said softly:

> I would guess it's been really emotionally draining for you. It's been probably very, very difficult because I've always been your rock just as much as you've always been mine.

Megan, with her own tears welling up in her eyes, reached over to take Dan's hand.

I could feel a cloud of heaviness come over Dan as he considered, for the first time, the shaping effects of his actions on Megan's life. However, not wanting to ease the weight of his anguish as it also came with a promise of a newfound sense of his accountability, I pressed on.

> Dan, this might be a difficult question....

Dan interrupted.

> That's okay. Go ahead and ask it.
>
> Okay, thanks Dan. I appreciate that. If you had to guess, knowing Megan as you do, what kind of effect or impact do you think it's had on Megan's sense of herself as a person to not have you there for her as you have always been?

Dan fell silent for what seemed to be a length of time given their conversational pace as he considered my question.

> I would have to think that it has been pretty demoralizing for her and really affected her sense of self-worth.

Dan's head was hanging low heading towards his chest. He glanced in Megan's direction; both their eyes were filled with tears.

> Megan, how is this going so far? How is Dan doing as a witness to your experience?
>> He is spot on. I had no idea that he understood what this was like for me.

While it was important for me to give Megan a chance to evaluate how the conversation was going, I wanted to build on the momentum of the conversation and the other-centered position that Dan was now able to take up.

> Megan, is it okay with you if I carry on a little longer speaking with Dan?

Megan responded enthusiastically:

> Yes, please!

I turned back to Dan, who seemed to be deep in contemplation.

> Dan, as you think about the effects these struggles in your relationship have brought to Megan's life – you used the words 'demoralizing' and 'draining' to describe the toll that it has taken on her life – is it okay with you that your pulling away from Megan has had that kind of impact on her?

Dan's reply was strong and unequivocal.

> No! It is not acceptable to me. Not at all!

Even in his soft-spoken manner, I could feel the force of his convictions behind his words.

> Why Dan? Why is it not okay with you? What was it that led you to speak with such conviction about your position that this is simply not acceptable?

Dan uttered with a heavy heart:

> Because I was the one who was always supposed to be there for her. No matter what.

> Can you help me understand this a bit better Dan? Why were you supposed to be the one that was to be there for her?
>
> Because I am her partner. Because I am her partner!

Dan's declared loudly as the force of conviction had clearly returned.

> Would I be right in guessing that you, somewhere along the way, made a promise to Megan that you would be there for her?

Dan and Megan gave each other a knowing glance as Dan took Megan's hand in his.

> Yes.

Dan spoke tenderly as Megan nodded while voicing a barely audible:

> Mhmm.
>
> Are you both remembering that moment right now?

They nodded in mutual consent.

> Can you tell me more about that promise Dan? Just how did you go about making this promise to Megan?
>
> It was very shortly before her mom's death. I'm a big comic book guy. That's an important background piece here. This is really relevant. She was crying to me and she was saying 'make it all go away, I don't want to deal with it, make it all go away.' I said to her, 'I can't do that love. I'm not Superman. I can't make it all go away. But I am a little like Batman. I can make it a little better.'

The significance of the Batman sweatshirt that Dan was wearing was now apparent to me as well as to them.

There was a brief pause in the conversation as they looked deeply into each other's eyes as if caught up in a shared memory of that moment. Megan began to weep.

> My dad had called me to tell me that my mom's cancer had spread to her brain...and the doctors only gave her a couple weeks. Dan was at work by that time. I called him and told him to come home. I'm surprised the operator at

159

> his work even knew who I was asking for because I was sobbing. I didn't even know if he even heard the words that came out. I was lying on the bed and I was just shaking because I was crying so hard.

Megan was sobbing even now recalling this to me.

> But after he came to me and said that he would be Batman for me, I knew that everything would be okay.

Megan fell into Dan's arms. The tenderness of this moment captured all of us and we sat together in a moment of honored silence.

> Dan, I couldn't help but notice that you are wearing a Batman sweatshirt today. That promise, Dan, for you to be a Batman for her, to be there for her, to make things better for her in a world that's not always going to be great to her, just how important is that to you?

Dan, still holding Megan in his arms, declared:

> It's the most important thing in the world to me.
> Over the last year, would you say that you have stepped away from your promise to be Batman for Megan?

It was Dan who was sobbing now.

> Yes. I've haven't been there for her and she has really been hurting. It's pretty disappointing.

Again, not wanting to take away from Dan's pain at realizing his own failures as a partner, I asked,

> And just how important is it to you to reclaim your role to be Batman for Megan?

Dan did not hesitate and the conviction in his voice returned.

> I would give up anything to reclaim that role.

Tears flowed freely between the three of us and no one dared to utter a word so as to not interrupt the beauty of what we had all been witness to on that day of our first session. I wondered to myself if this, in and of itself, would defy the destined dissolution of their relationship. Knowing that our time would soon be up, I broke the silence.

> There is so much more that I want to ask you about but we are almost out of time. Still, I want to thank you both for the tenderness of your words and for letting me be a witness to such a painfully beautiful moment in your lives. Before we part, could I ask you both to consider one thing between now and the time that we meet again? We talked today, mostly to you Dan, about the effects of your shared struggles and that your own actions have had on Megan and how she experiences herself as a person and a partner. Dan and Megan, would you be willing think about what you would hope for most in terms of how you want each other to feel when they are in your presence? For example, what messages do you want your thoughts, your feelings, and your actions to send each other about how you feel about them as a person? Would that be okay?

Megan and Dan wholeheartedly agreed to take up my invitation to consider this.

Session Two

Megan, Dan, and I met for our second meeting one month later. I had some time before our session, so I decided to review my notes from our previous meeting. I found myself being swept up all over again by the many painful and tender expressions that were shared between them. As I was walking to the waiting room, I remembered the image of them sitting apart, starting at their phone and the alarm I felt at the lack of any liveliness between them. I admit to having felt a bit anxious at what I would find this time. As I peered around the corner just before entering the waiting room, any concerns that I might have had faded away. Megan and Dan were sitting on a love seat, their arms outstretched toward each other, and deep in conversation. I even had to get their attention as they didn't seem to notice me enter the waiting room.

I began the session by asking Megan and Dan if it would be okay if I offered a bit of retelling of what it was that we talked about when we last met and some of the significant conclusions that they came to about each other and their relationship. As I was reading through the notes of the conversation, Megan and Dan were caught by surprise several times at their words, saying things such as, "Did we really say that?" and "Dan really understands me much more than I had thought", but what they really wanted to talk about was Dan's promise to be batman for Megan.

Dan said:

> That really got me. It was on my mind every day for the past month. More like, the promise had a hold on me. It wouldn't let go of me. Although the promise transformed into something more. Not just to be batman but a desire for her to feel loved by me.

> The promise wouldn't let go of you, Dan. That's an interesting way to say that. Would you mind if I asked you both a few questions about this? Would that be a good place for us to start?

Megan and Dan nodded in agreement.

> This might seem like a backward way to ask this but can I ask you, Megan, to give an account of the ways that you saw Dan living up to his promise to be Batman for you since we last met? I know it has been awhile so, if it is easier, you might just wish to think about the last week or so.

> Sure! I am up for that. Dan was on the hot seat last time so it is only fair that it is my turn to speak.
>
> Okay, thanks Megan. As you look back over the past week or so as a witness to Dan's actions, what were some of the ways that you noticed Dan acting on his promise to be Batman for you?

Megan rattled off a list of a few things, before settling on one that seemed most significant to her.

> I have this really disgusting gravy boat. This is the way he'll describe it, 'disgusting!'
>
> Did I hear you right? Did you say a 'gravy boat?',

I was curious to know why Megan would nominate this as a particularly important verification of Dan's love for her.

> Megan continued.

> That's right, a gravy boat. It's a hippopotamus, actually.

Dan couldn't help but chime in.

> It's horrifying. The gravy comes out the hippo's mouth. The hippo literally vomits gravy. Words cannot describe how disgusting it is.
>
> "Wow, thanks for that image Dan," I quipped as laughter filled the room.
>
> Okay, Megan so why is it that you nominated this hippo gravy boat as a moment when you witnessed Dan acting on his desire for you to feel loved?

Megan's sarcasm quickly subsided as her tone became more somber.

> It was my favorite thing growing up. My mom said she threw it away. When we were going through her cupboards to clean stuff out when she got sick, I found the hippo. So, then I took it and put it in protective custody. Dan told me a long time ago that we could only use it when we were just the two of us, but he was opposed to us using it as a dinner party gravy boat.

Laughter returned to the room as I asked:

> Okay, so now it is a dinner party hippo gravy boat. Do I have that right?

Megan replied:

> Yes, we're having his parents over for Thanksgiving tomorrow, so I was like, 'oh, I want to go buy a gravy boat.' But they were just too expensive. I hate spending money on things, and how often do you really use a gravy boat. I was complaining to Dan about the cost and do you know what he said? He said, 'We can use the hippo.' I couldn't believe my ears. I was banned from using this hippo, especially in front of his mom, who was coming to dinner tomorrow.

While the symbolic significance of the hippo gravy boat and its connection to Megan's mom was clear to me, I was not yet sure if it had dawned on Dan just yet, so I pressed further.

> "Okay Megan, when Dan shocked you and said that you can finally use the hippo in front of his mother, of all people, what message was he sending you about how he feels about you? What was he telling you about how he felt about you in that moment when he said, 'all right you can use the hippo'?" Megan's voice fell soft again, in what I took to be her attempt to dignify this with gravity.
>
> That he really cared about me, and he cared about my ridiculous emotional attachment to a hippo gravy boat. And he was willing to sacrifice his parents for it.

Wanting to extend the significance of Dan's action in this matter as far as possible, I asked: "I'm wondering Megan, is there any significance about Dan's acceptance of your relationship with this hippo given that his parents were coming?"

Megan answered:

> Yes, because I've often felt that his parents were more important to him than me, that he cared more about their opinion than mine. So, caring more about what I wanted and what I liked over what his parents would like was really important to me.
>
> Megan, what do you think he might have been saying about your importance to him in relation to his parents?
>
> That he cared more about my thoughts and feelings than theirs. I felt as if I was gaining more importance than them in his life.

Wanting to extend the significance of this realization on Megan's part I asked:

> And what did it offer you, Megan, when Dan told you, through his actions, that you and your desires were more important than his parents?

Megan was quiet for a moment as her eyes peered up and over to the right as if she was searching for the right words.

> Look, I get parents are an important part of your life. But it was just bothering me that in big life decisions, he would always have to confirm everything with them even after he discussed it with me. I wanted our relationship to become more of a partnership without parents' influence so much...not without their influence, but that our relationship would be the priority.

Megan once again fell silent for a moment as tears began to well up in her eyes. Nevertheless, she continued:

> So having him accept me and say, 'you can have this hippo. I don't really care what my mom thinks. If she doesn't want to use it then she doesn't have to put gravy on her turkey' It was validating that my importance was there and that we are an independent unit from his parents.
>
> As you look back now from this very moment with all that you have said up to this point, what might Dan's actions of accepting the hippo gravy boat suggest about your place in his life?

Megan's voice grew soft as tears fell softly down her face.

> That I'm number one in his heart. That I am number one in his heart.

While her voice was soft, her words were declarative. I pressed on:

> Megan, this feeling of being number one in his heart, what is that offering you in terms of how you feel about yourself and your relationship with Dan?

Megan's voice grew strong again.

> I think it's security. I just feel more secure in life and where we are as a couple. It makes me feel that I have somebody in my corner who accepts my very extreme weirdness at times. It just made me feel more comfortable being me. Him accepting the hippo gravy boat was accepting me.

The conversation with Megan had yielded something entirely unexpected. I am not sure if either of them were aware of the significance of all of this at the time, but somehow Dan's offering of something seemingly so simple as using the hippo gravy boat was transformed into a powerful witness of his love that led Megan to conclude that she was number one in his heart. And while we had already spent almost the entire session talking about this one event, I turned to Dan in hopes that he might connect his actions to his growing awareness of the special relationship between Megan and her mom.

> Dan, having been a witness to everything Megan has said here today, is it important to you that she be able to hold on to the significance and memories of the hippo?

Dan's response was immediate.

> Yes. It really is.
>
> Why, Dan? Can you help me understand why it is important to you that she hold on to her relationship with the hippo?

Dan tenderly said:

> Megan's mom is really important to her. The hippo is a tie between her and her mom. She doesn't have a whole lot of those things left anymore, so this one's important. It means a lot.

Hearing his response, Megan once began to cry. Wanting to know more about what Megan's tears might be on behalf of, I asked:

> Megan, is there something about what Dan said that was particularly moving that brought the tears to the surface?

Through her sobbing, Megan said haltingly:

> It's just... It's just... The holiday season was my mom's favorite time of year, so I have a love/hate relationship with it. It was just nice to hear that he was willing to accept my weird things so I can still have those connections to my mom.

I asked tenderly:

> Megan, what feelings come to you now, as you hear Dan saying that he was connecting the using of the hippo as a way of acknowledging and maintaining your relationship with your mom?
>
> Unfortunately, he didn't get that long to know my mom. But my mom really loved the hippo, so it's like he understands how close and how similar my mom and I were. And saying no to the hippo was like saying 'no' to my mom and saying 'no' to my past.
>
> Before this conversation today, did you know that he understood or appreciated the connection between the hippo and your relationship with your mom?

Megan's tears continued to flow as she uttered an almost inaudible:

> No.
>
> What is it like for you to know that he can now appreciate that?
>
> It's a little bit great and a little bit heartbreaking. I wish he could've known my mom longer so that he could see our shared craziness. Because my mom and I, if you saw us together, you could totally tell we were related. We were the same bit of crazy.

Wanting to return the conversation to Dan, I repeated Megan's words "the same bit of crazy" and asked:

> Dan, what do you think about this crazy in Megan?
>
> I get it. I've sort of known that that little bit of crazy comes from her mom the whole time. Just the little bit that I did get to know, it was always amazing to me how similar Renee was to Megan.

Dan then turned to Megan and said through his tears:

I know there are lots of little things like that that you associate with your mom around the holidays and that it is a tough time for you. I know that. It's the reason that I never, never, ever even approach the topic of the snowman dishes even though they're a little dorky.

Megan said with a tender laugh:

They're amazing.

Why are they amazing? I'm going to ask you that question, Dan. Why do you think that Megan would say that the snowman dishes are amazing?

Dan reached over to take Megan's hand before saying softly:

The snowman dishes *are* amazing.... Even though they are so loud and bright, they are beautiful because they were her mom's, and her mom loved and adored these snowman dishes. Megan fought tooth and nail to get these snowman dishes from her sisters. After her mom's death, the first time ever, we're going to use these snowman dishes this Thanksgiving.

Megan, I heard Dan saying that the snowman dishes are beautiful. I am just wondering what was it like for you to hear him acknowledge their beauty?

Megan was quiet, as if trying to take in Dan's words.

I always thought he hated them, so it's kind of sweet to hear that he actually thinks they're beautiful. For years, they've just been kind of hauled back and forth in boxes between here and there and everywhere. We've never used them. So, it's really great. Especially because they are so ridiculously bright-colored for winter dishes. I would never want a plain, boring dish.

Is that 'the little bit of crazy' that you inherited from your mom coming through?

Yes, It's a little bit of crazy. It's more fun.

I'm wondering, Dan, if there's something about Megan's little bit of crazy that drew you to her?

Dan said with a smile:

"I love it." It's one of those things that endeared me to her early on when we were dating...her little bit of crazy. In fact, there is a Doctor Seuss quote that we put on our wedding invitation....

And triumphantly, and in unison, Megan and Dan said:

> Life is a little weird. We're all a little weird. You have to find somebody whose weirdness matches yours, and call it a mutual weirdness, and call it love.

Once again, our time was almost up. While the significance of all that they had accomplished over the past month was clearly apparent to me, I wanted to give Megan and Dan a chance to "speak" it into being.

> I am just sitting here thinking back to the first time that you came to see me and the pain that you brought with you. The feelings of resentment, the coldness, the name calling. And most of all, the feeling of having to live with the loss of your best friendship. I don't bring this up to take you back there in any way, but rather to give you both a moment to reflect on how far you have come in such a short time. And this is just our second meeting together. If you were to take a moment and pause and just take it all in..., what feelings do you have for each other and for your relationship that you didn't have before?

The tears returned in full force to both of them.

> I am just so grateful to have my Dan, my best friend, my Batman back.
>
> Would you say, Megan, that he is back in the same way that he was before or is he back in a different way?
>
> He is back in a way that is more than I could have ever hoped for. I guess I don't just have my best friend back, I have even more.

Megan's words brought a tender smile to Dan's face.

> I am really proud of Megan and of our relationship. We not only brought it back but we moved it forward in ways that we never thought possible.

Even though we decided that this would be our last session, I asked Megan and Dan if they would be willing to meet with me one last time, not as therapy, but to interview them as consultants about what they found most helpful or interesting about our work together and see if there was anything that they would want other couples to know about who were experiencing similar struggles. Megan and Dan were more than happy to agree such a consultation.

We met one month later. I began the meeting by reflecting on where things were when we started, the distance, coldness, and quiet resentment and disregard that had come between their best friendship. I marveled aloud at how quickly and seemingly easily things turned around for them and asked if they might help me out by making some guesses as to what it was in our conversations together that made that possible.

Dan responded first.

> You know, if I had to guess, it had something to do with the way you asked questions. You almost never asked me to speak directly about my experience, which I have to admit was a surprise at first. You come to a counselor thinking that they are going to ask each person to talk about what the relationship is like to each of them. But you didn't do that. From the get-go, you asked me to think and speak about Megan's experience of this relationship and our struggles together. And I guess that really made a difference for me. Before, I was so caught up on me, and my experience, that I never really considered what it was like for Megan.

As I turned to Megan, she looked deep in thought.

> I agree with what Dan said but there is something more, at least for me. As you were asking Dan to speak about my experience, I was surprised at how closely he had been listening to me. I had no idea that he knew what all of this has been like for me. That was probably the most meaningful thing to me...the thing that made the biggest difference for me.
>
> It is interesting that you say that, Megan and Dan. Is it possible that by being invited into a position of a witness of the other that it gives people the means to get beyond their own experience and into the experience of the other? And one more thing, I remember how you both expressed knowing so little about what your struggles were actually like for the other and how you both took up the invitation to be a witness to each other's experience. Is it possible that other couples would long for this...long to be invited into an intimate appreciation of the experience of their partners when they are in the midst of the perils and struggles of life?

Megan and Dan had much more to say about this but let me end with this enthusiastic comment by Megan:

> Hell yes! I found it much more interesting when Dan was speaking about my experience than if you had asked me to tell you about myself. My deepest, most secret longing in life is to know that me and my experience is known by Dan. And he knew me in ways that I didn't even know were possible.

Now it was Dan who fell into Megan's arms as he whispered:

> I am sorry that it took me so long, my love. I am back and always will be.

A Surprise Meeting

The story doesn't end here. It was a warm spring day, 18 months later. I was at an outdoor market. I saw my favorite vendor and made an immediate a beeline in hopes that there still might be a loaf of my favorite bread left for sale. As I got to the line, I looked up and saw Megan and Dan standing right in front of me. After we exchanged excited and warm greetings, Megan moved to the side revealing a stroller and said:

> Tom, there is someone we want to introduce you to. Do you remember when we came to see you almost two years ago that we said that we didn't want to bring a baby into this relationship? Well, here she is. And we couldn't be more pleased.

Chapter 7

"MAYBE WE ARE OKAY"
Contemporary Narrative Therapy in the Time of Trump

Travis Heath

A quick glance at the clock adjacent to the bed reveals that the time is 6:37 am. I peek over at my partner who is also lying awake with a look of deep contemplation on her face. As she glances at me, her lips refuse to release the grimace of concern. At this moment, I know it isn't just a dream that is trying to nip at the heels of my waking life.

> "How can this happen?" she asks.
> I wish I had a good answer for you.
> "What will we tell our daughters?" she persists, with tears welling up in her eyes.
> How are we going to raise these girls in a world like this?

Most often I could muster up some kind of answer for even the most difficult of questions she had thrown my way in our over 17 years of partnership. On this morning, however, I have none. All I can do is extend my arms gesturing for her to accept my cocoon of comfort. Neither of us are able to console the other. We cry together.

The duties of the world beckon as we hear our five-year-old daughter stirring. Our inertia is quickly disrupted as she makes her way into our room.

The remainder of the morning seems unremarkable, albeit melancholy, as I slog through my academic duties at Metropolitan State University of

DOI: 10.4324/9781003226543-9

Denver. Around lunchtime a student whom I know well enters my office. Almost before he sits down, he begins sobbing as though a two-liter bottle of soda had been shaken vigorously and then the cap removed.

> "I don't know how much longer I'll be here," he yowls, fearful that the President-elect would soon send United States Immigration and Customs Enforcement officers to remove him or his family to a country where his ancestors once resided but where he has never set foot. Any consoling words I might offer seem inadequate. I hope my somewhat steady and familiar presence might prove to be suffice. But the truth is, nothing feels like enough.

My mind darts this way and that as I try to project some semblance of the professor my students have come to know over time. But the thought of Donald Trump as President buzzes around my consciousness like that fly one can never quite shoo.

The clock turns 7 pm and I quickly make my way out of my academic surroundings to my car en route to my private practice office where I meet with one person at the end of my teaching day. While some might think the act of therapy to be an exhausting one, especially after a full day of teaching, I have nearly always been energized by it. It almost serves as a refuge of sorts.

I exhale deeply with a feeling of relief that I am heading to this safe haven. I feel a slight jolt as the back tire of my car hits the curb, something I rarely do, as I attempt to parallel park. It is apparent this distraction that has followed me all day is still very much in tow. Walking up the steps at the front of the building, still seven minutes until our conversation is scheduled to commence, I see Jane sitting in the lonely and empty waiting area reading a magazine. We have been in conversation with each other, meeting bi-weekly, for over three months. As we are walking together up the second flight of stairs to the top floor of the old mansion where my office is located, she is uncharacteristically reserved. I unlock the door and flip on the lights. She wanders to the two big windows at the front of the office that look out over the city. As I am setting my bag down and getting out my pen and paper, before even sitting down, she earnestly asks me a question that invites a ping of anxiety in my chest.

> You voted for Hillary, didn't you?

The question doesn't quite feel accusatory, but the words travel crisply enough through the air to stir up a bit of tension.

My mind is racing trying to prepare a suitable response. I can hear in my mind's ear the professors who administered much of my formal training prohibiting any self-disclosure and instead advising responses of this sort, "That's an interesting question. I wonder what makes you ask that?" I shake off such a suggestion and almost chuckle out loud knowing that she knows me well enough at this stage to call bullshit on such a charade.

I pause, trying to consult other mentors and prized elders who have helped me along my path to becoming a therapist. I know what I have to do.

> "Yeah, I did," I respond, endeavoring to strike a tone of openness blended with steadfastness.

Her head drops and she snickers.

> Yeah, I figured you did.

A number of poorly thought out and what would ultimately be unproductive questions cycle through my mind, the kind that political dichotomies seem to only accentuate.

> You figured I did? What the fuck is that supposed to mean?!? You don't even really know me!

I paused and those questions, which fortunately never left the confines of my mind, give rise to a hint of curiosity.

I say aloud in a tone that I hope she will recognize as respectful from our previous conversations:

> Do you mind if I ask you a question?

After pausing for a few seconds, she replies:

> No, go ahead.

I query in a gentle voice:

> Might I ask who you voted for?

She seems to assume a guarded and almost amused posture in regard to my question. A skeptical smile overtakes her face as though she foresees the risk of going down this road together.

> "Trump!" she announces.

At this moment, a chasm is opening up in the room. It threatens our relationship the way a thunderstorm does when it's approaching quickly across the horizon. It feels like the direction of our work and the relationship we share is now dependent on how we handle this admission that we have been crossing enemy lines for the better part of the last three months. Pondering the seditiousness of such an act excites me and momentarily takes me in a different direction.

> "Wow!" I exclaim. "Don't you think this is amazing?"

She cocks her head in utter confusion seemingly baffled.
I say with a bit of a twinkle in my eye:

> May I ask you a question?

She nods her assent.

> Do you like me as a human being?
> "Of course I do," she replies without hesitation.
> "May I share something with you?" I continue.

She gestures for me to continue with a quick nod of her head.

> I like you, too.

A momentary silence falls over the room before I add:

> Do you think our country would currently endorse such a relationship?

She directs a somewhat befuddled gaze at me in response before asking:

> What do you mean?

I heard an increasing urgency in my tone of voice.

> Do you know many Trump supporters and Hillary supporters out in the world who share this kind of relationship?

After a hearty chuckle, she replies:

> Not many.

It is as if we both need to pause for a few seconds to think about how preposterous this all seems given the current state of our union. Perhaps we are also puzzling over just how ridiculous this particular arrangement appears on the surface. A 36-year-old, agnostic, brown, dreadlocked therapist with tattoos peeking out of his sleeves working with a 58-year-old, white, born again Christian woman. This isn't exactly the kind of relationship typically discussed in psychotherapy textbooks.

I ask:

> How are we pulling this off? I mean, is this real, or do you think we are fooling ourselves?

Jane justifies our collaboration:

> Well, my friend Karen said she had panic attacks so bad that she was pulling out her hair and after coming to see you for a few months they went away. And I trust her more than anyone.
>
> Did that trust somehow find its way into our relationship?

Jane says with a hint of trepidation:

> Well, I mean, she warned me that you were... no offense, weird. Like, not the kind of person you might expect to see when you go to a therapist.
>
> "That's a relief," I quip. "I always get concerned when people start thinking I'm normal."

We share a laugh that seems to ease the tension. While humor is a seemingly welcome distraction, tension circles back like the villain in a horror movie that leaps up from its grave to grab you by the ankle making you regret you thought it was dead.

As the silence grows, I take some time to mull over the work we have been doing together, perhaps to distract myself from the discomfiture. When Jane first arrived in my office nearly three months earlier, she had just been released from a psychiatric hospital. Her hospital stay was precipitated by an explosive argument with her husband of 28 years that left her feeling as though she no longer wished to live. Shame and confusion about the worthwhileness of her life followed her into our first meeting and were convincing her that she had no purpose in living. In our last meeting two weeks before, Jane celebrated what she described as "breakthroughs," the most important of which she detailed as a rediscovery of her relationship with God. I feel my lips begin to take the shape of a smile as I ponder the vivacity of our previous meeting. Jane's energy was certainly something I had come to really appreciate about her. The reminiscence doesn't last long as I experience a smash-cut back to the conversation at hand.

> "Jane, is it alright if I ask you something else," I say, endeavoring to assume a stance of invitation.

She nods in agreement.

> Have you known I was someone who would likely vote for Hillary for a while or is this a realization you came to recently?

She starts chuckling as if to draw our attention to the naivety of my question.

> Well, you don't exactly seem like the type of guy who would vote for Trump.

I return the chuckle.

> It's that obvious, huh?

She doesn't miss a beat.

It's pretty obvious, yeah.

"May I ask you another question about this?" I continue, a bit nervous to hear her response.

She again nods affirmatively.

Might I ask why you decided to go down this road with me in the first place? Would it be fair to say that was taking quite a risk?

Jane pauses for a few seconds, her face assuming a more serious and pensive expression.

I was in such a bad spot that I didn't know where else to go. I was desperate.

I take a moment to metabolize her response before asking:

Once you got here and we began our work together, what was it that made you trust I would take good care of your stories even despite the fact that we might have been placed by the world into two different political camps?

She responds with conviction:

Oh, I didn't even really think about that too much. I got the sense that you cared about me, like beyond just a way to make money. It was like the whole politics thing didn't matter.

The last sentence Jane utters sticks to me like a piece of gum one steps on that won't come off the bottom of one's shoe. The whole politics thing didn't matter? I begin quietly asking myself a series of questions, something that happens to me often when in conversation with someone almost as if I'm trying to cycle through questions to find the best one to ask. How does it come to be that politics don't matter in a relationship? How is it that they might not matter at one point and come to matter again at another? As these questions run sprints through my consciousness, I can see Jane becoming a little restless.

Jane, given that you said politics didn't matter when you first came to see me, is it okay if I ask how they found their way into our meeting this evening?

179

This question causes Jane more pause than most of the questions I have asked her.

> "Well," she began, "it kind of feels like politics are involved in everything right now. It's pretty much like all that people are talking about. I guess there was just no way to avoid it."

Avoid is such a tricky word, I think to myself. It pesters me for a few seconds. I continue:

> How did you come to understand that politics should be avoided in conversation?
> It's like they say, avoid all talk of religion and politics, right?

My eyes light up a bit as I say:

> Yeah, I've heard that old saying, too. Hey Jane, do you think that's an accurate statement? Like, is it one we should live by or would you prefer to live by another credo?
> I haven't really given it much thought, to be honest. I guess it's a good way to go.
> "Would it be alright if I shared something with you," I ask hopefully.
> Sure.
> "I'm fairly certain my field abides by this idea that religion and politics are often subjects that should be for the most part avoided, too" I explain. "Why do you think it is that both of us chose to break this rule in our conversation tonight? Did you have any sense that there might be value in doing so?"
> I'm really not sure.

I follow-up.

> As we are talking about it now are you finding it to be of any value or do you think it would serve us better to go in another direction?

She thinks diligently about my query before reaching her solution.

> Now that you mention it, I feel like we are being more real with each other. It's also like rebellious or something.

I am now finding it hard to conceal my excitement. The thought of therapy as an act of rebellion is intoxicating.

> What would you say we might be rebelling against?
> "You know, just this idea that two people would be so different because of who they voted for," Jane asserts. "Maybe we're not that different. Or even if we are different in certain ways maybe that is only on the surface."
> Do you think it feels unfair that we have basically only been given two options?

Without hesitating Jane emphatically replies:

> Yes!

The amount of certitude in Jane's voice inspires confidence in me to pursue the conversation a bit further.

> Jane, would you say that the political category that you are squeezed into sometimes fails to fit for you?
> Oh yeah! There are definitely things I don't like about what the Republicans believe. And just so you know, it's not like I agree with everything Trump does or says, either.

A bit of defensiveness seems to settle over the room. While uncomfortable, I wonder if it's the kind of defensiveness that might have the ability to take us somewhere important, though I am not sure exactly where quite yet.

> I just had a wild idea, Jane. Is it alright if I share it with you?

She nods her assent.

> Do you suppose we might be in the process of creating a third category right now?

She replies with a perplexed look:

> What do you mean?

Anticipating this might be her response, I am ready with a follow-up question.

> Through our conversation today are we carving out something that is neither Trump nor Hillary? Are we perhaps creating something that transcends the two options we have been given to define our political identities - a third way forward?

It becomes increasingly clear given the grimace on Jane's face that my question is leaving her feeling somewhat taken aback. After taking some time to consider my proposal, she declares:

> Well, I still would have voted for Trump if that's what you're asking.

Steeling for potential further discomfort, I ask:

> Earlier you said having this conversation is inviting us to be more real with one another and might be an act of rebellion, right?

Jane gives an affirmative nod.

> Would you say rebels typically adopt already existing ideologies or do they yearn to create ideologies of their own?

She states confidently:

> Rebels create something new.

I ask in a curiously soft voice:

> Do you have some sense of what these two rebels might be creating together tonight?
> "That's a tough question. I'm not even sure," she says with puzzlement settling on her brow.

I look up and notice the clock just a few ticks away from 8:30 pm, our signal to put this conversation to rest. Jane and I make an agreement that we will live with this question of what a Trump rebel and Hillary rebel might be creating together between now and our next conversation. It feels like an admittedly awkward end to a conversation the likes of which neither of us had ever had. However, in the past we often agreed to live with questions between meetings, so my proposal was not out of the ordinary. As I walk with Jane down the winding mansion stairs to the front door, I can already feel doubt in tow. We say goodbye to one another, and I collapse onto one of the waiting room couches where I stay for several minutes staring at the tangled mass of colors on the abstract painting on the wall 15-feet away in the now abandoned mansion.

I collect myself, lock the front door, and make my way to the car. On the way there, I shiver just a little bit and notice the water vapor in my breath is now visible. I exhale deeply a couple of times just so I can get a good look at the fog I can create through my own breathing, perhaps hoping the fog will reveal an answer to this elusive riddle. This winter ritual had always brought an odd sense of comfort to me ever since I was a young boy.

I climb in the driver's seat of the car, start the engine, and drive away. It doesn't take long to notice that doubt is riding shotgun and primed to start the process of interrogating me.

What will my narrative therapy friends think about this? Am I selling out by working with a Trump supporter? Am I practicing the wrong kind of 'social justice?'

I notice a look of consternation mixed with contemplation as I catch a quick glance of my face in the rearview mirror. I can feel rebuttals brewing in my soul.

What is social justice, anyway? Might I need to start anew and refashion my understanding of social justice? Have I been adhering to a canonized version of social justice that could engage in the same damaging habit that social justice movements had set out to try and avoid in the first place?

These questions were constant companions for the week in advance of my next meeting with Jane. Any resolutions, however, remained elusive.

Upon our next meeting before I was able to ask anything, Jane states:

> I've been thinking about the question you asked. You know, the one about a third category or whatever that we might be making together?

I nod in eager but also anxious anticipation as to where this might lead.

> "Well," Jane proposes, "I think we're creating a human category."

I proceed with a tone of urgent curiosity.

> Is it alright if I ask you a little bit more about this category, Jane?

She nods her assent.

> Would it be right to say that the way these political parties have taken shape in our country can strip us of our humanity?
> "Yes," Jane replies with a fire burning warmer in her eyes.
> It's like we don't even see people as people anymore.
> You know, Jane, I was thinking about that this week. If you had to venture a guess, would you guess that my therapist friends are Hillary supporters or Trump supporters?

A cackle ejected itself from Jane's mouth.

> "That's easy," she says. "Hillary all the way."
> And if you had to guess what they might say about me seeing you, what might be your guess?

Jane pauses, appearing to really contemplate the question.

> "I don't know," she says, "maybe that you're crazy to see me or something like that?"
> "Unfortunately, I'm not sure you're that far off," I reply. "And to be honest, I'm afraid I could have said something similar."

This admission seems to stir something in Jane. I'm struggling to tell if she is being visited by hurt, anger, or something else altogether. I decide to let the moment breathe for a while.

I re-engage by asking:

> What bits of humanity am I getting to see in you that I might otherwise have missed out on had I not broken ranks with my group?

Jane's tone feels more vulnerable as she responds:

> That I'm a caring person. That I will go to the ends of the earth for the people I love.

Jane pauses and begins to cry.

> That I love all of God's creatures, even those different from me.

Jane begins to sob more intensely and places her face in her palms. She then waves her left hand quickly as if to try and shake off the tears. She declares:

> My dad was a Republican. After he died, I felt a kind of responsibility to carry this on. Not that I do it just for him, but I know it was important to him. I know he wouldn't be pleased with everything about Trump. But I was forced into picking him, you know! I mean, what were my other options? I don't want to let my dad down. It's not like Trump was all bad or something, but I just felt trapped by the whole thing.

The room is overtaken by silence. It feels as if Jane might be baring a part of her soul that she hasn't previously revealed in our conversations together. I start to feel just how deep Jane's relationship with the political ideas of her family runs. Questions start cycling through my head. What if this is less about ideology and more about feeling connected to family? How much might this be informing her identity? If it is informing her identity, does a criticism of Trump or Republican politicians start to feel like a personal criticism of her? I lean back in my chair, rub my right temple with my thumb and index finger, and think deeply, almost meditatively, about these ideas. After what seemed to me to be an inordinately lengthy silence, a question emerges from the depth of my being.

> Might I apologize, Jane, for having prejudged you based on who you voted for?
>
> "What do you mean?" Jane replies, her eyes straining with perplexity.
>
> Is it possible I might have insulted a part of you that is deeply connected to your family and whom you know yourself to be?

Jane shakes her head from left to right in a determined fashion and declares:

> No, I never felt insulted by you.

Although I feel Jane has exonerated me, I still wonder if something else needs to be addressed:

> Do you sometimes feel that people who have different political beliefs from you insult this part of your heart and soul that is connected to your family?
> "Yeah, sometimes," she admits.
> When they do this would you say they are missing the part of you that is caring, loyal, and loves all God's creatures as you were telling me earlier?

Her nodding affirms my query.
I continue as if my questions are now falling into a bit of a rhythm:

> What are the consequences for our living when we miss these parts of one another because of politics?

Jane listens intently to my question. It's as if she has an answer but is reluctant to let it leave the confines of her mind and utter it aloud.

> The consequence,

she says pausing for 10 or so seconds before apprehensively finishing the sentence,

> is hate.

Trying to assume a steady tone, I ask:

> When we are up against hate is that when the humanness you told me about at the beginning of our meeting is perhaps of most importance?

A tear begins to make its slow descent down Jane's left cheek. She nods her head in affirmation. Fearing that words could get in the way of this moment, I make a quick pact with myself to allow the heavy but seemingly important silence to linger.

Jane looks up slowly and says with her voice breaking up:

> I don't hate you. I want you to know that.

I nod in solidarity with Jane and reply:

> I don't hate you, either. Quite the contrary, actually.

A tiny smile begins to break through the heaviness on Jane's face. I ask:

> How have we together not allowed hate to strip us of our humanity in here?
> By having a conversation with each other,

she replies, her voice now carrying a little more hope.

> It's dangerous to think you know someone just because of a group they are in or who they voted for. And give them a chance because you might actually like them.

The smile on Jane's face grows a bit wider.

Feeling the warmth, the way one does when sitting by an open fire after coming in from the cold, I query:

> Jane, do you think we might be experiencing the third category of humanness you talked about earlier in our relationship right now?

She nods affirmatively.

> Yeah, I would say so.

In this moment, part of me wants to bask in the warm glow that experiencing humanness together was bestowing upon us. Another part of me was pleading not to be lulled to sleep by this, insisting that there was more work to be done. In that spirit, I ask:

> Do you think it might be important for us to continue to stand up for this third category of humanness in our living out there in the world or should this just be a project for in here?

After a deep sigh, Jane responds:

> I think it will be hard to do it out there. It feels safe to talk about this in here. I know that you won't judge me or think badly of me.

Feeling the need to persist, I ask:

> Do you think this conversation might have a spirit to it that could travel with us?

Jane looks somewhat confused.

> I'm not sure what you mean.

Collecting myself, I try again.

> What could our country out there learn from our relationship right now?

Jane indicates by subtly nodding that my question is now making more sense. She begins:

> That there is some kind of middle ground. Actually, more than a middle ground. That people who vote for different candidates can like each other. Like if someone out in the world said something bad about you, I would set them straight. I would have your back. You're a good person.

I notice myself feeling moved by Jane's words. The feeling of a lump in my throat seems more obstructive.

> Jane, I want you to know how much your words mean to me. Thank you. And I also want you to know that I would have your back out in the world, too. Do you suppose that might be the spirit of what we're talking about here that we could take out into the world? If you take the time to create humanness with a person, even a person who has been placed in a different political category than you, that they might have a back worth protecting?

Jane says with a certain measure of assurance:

> Yes, I think that's right.

I add in a playful but honest tone:

> I mean, it's safe to say that our differences still exist, right? We didn't get rid of those?

Returning the playful smile, she replies:

> Oh, no! They definitely still exist.

I continue, knowing there might be some risk in moving this direction:

> Have we discovered that part of this work involves learning to sit alongside differences rather than to eradicate them?
> What do you mean?

I continue without losing momentum:

> Have you noticed that often when two people of different political persuasions get together, they spend all their time together trying to convince the other one to come over to their side?
> "Yeah, ain't that the truth," she says vociferously.
> Would you say we're not doing that?

I follow-up.

> We're living with difference rather than trying to change it?

She contemplates in what appears to be a rather deep fashion for a few seconds before uttering:

> Uh-huh.

I ask:

> Do you suppose that the fact we don't agree in some ways politically could actually add something to our relationship and the work we're doing that we couldn't access if we had the same political beliefs? Might it actually in a weird way be helping us locate a humanness in one another we might not find if our beliefs were similar?

189

She replies with a smile:

> Yeah, you know, I was thinking about that. Facing all of this with you makes me feel more hopeful. I was telling my husband that I feel like I can overcome differences with other people in my life. And this may sound like naïve or something, but if we can do this together, why can't other people?

Feeling energized, I ask:

> Jane, I'm just guessing here so I know I could be wrong, but might that be an example of the very spirit we're creating together in this room traveling outside into the world?
> Huh,

she says, with all the curiosity of a scientist whose fortune had prepared their mind when stumbling over an important discovery.

> I guess that's right.

I continue, knowing our time is close to expiration:

> Jane, I know that our pattern has been to leave with a question for both of us to live with between meetings. Would it be alright if I advance one and you tell me whether or not it's a good one? If it's not, perhaps we can locate a different one?

She nods for me to continue. I oblige.

> What if between now and the next time we meet we keep an eye out for the way humanness is finding us in the world, most especially with people that we might otherwise not see eye-to-eye with?

Jane asserts:

> Yeah, I like that.

It's not uncommon for a question like the one I posed to Jane to follow me in between meetings. This particular question, however, seems to stalk me. I find it hiding in the broad daylights in plain sight where I might never have expected.

On a Tuesday in the late fall, I wander into a coffee shot to get some tea. As I'm waiting in line, I hear two men in front of me espousing the merits of what electing Trump will do for United States' economy. I almost immediately feel enveloped by suspicion and contempt. Before either reaches full maturity, though, I feel the question I shared with Jane in our last meeting intervene. I find myself wondering about the lives of the two men in front of me. How did they come to support Trump? Was it a family connection like Jane's or did it happen in a different way? Did they know I didn't vote for Trump? Would we be able to have a conversation and maybe even develop a friendship despite this political divide?

> Sir, may I take your order?
> I hear a voice say almost optionally seemingly from afar as though I am in a lucid dream. "Sir?"

The voice repeats itself a bit louder. This shakes me out of my reveries and back into everyday reality. I look up and notice there is 15-feet between me and the cashier and a slew of impatient patrons standing in line behind me. I sheepishly approach the counter and place my order. As I collect my tea and head back to my car I wonder if this question is in dogged pursuit of Jane in the same way it's shadowing me.

Two weeks later, Jane and I meet again. Jane's being seems to assume a more meditative posture. This strikes me as being different and engages my curiosity.

> Jane, I know I'm just guessing and could be wrong, but is it possible that a certain serenity has accompanied you into the room tonight?

A quiet and persistent smile makes its way onto Jane's lips.

> I knew you would catch that.
> Can you help me understand a little bit better what exactly we're reeling in here?

I return the smile while making the motion of a fisherman reeling in a weighty but as yet unknown catch.

> It's like the anxiety has started melting away or something.

Jane's eyes hint at some unsolved mystery.

> We haven't even been talking about anxiety at all these last couple of meetings, but somehow, it's just disappeared. I mean, it was already starting to go down, but now it's like...*gone*.
>
> What's your sense of why it's disappeared, Jane? Do you think it has anything to do with what we've been talking about in our conversations or perhaps something different altogether?

I lean forward eagerly awaiting her response.

> I don't know. Do you think the anxiety could have had something to do with all of this?

Jane appears dumbfounded by the possibility. Having worked with me long enough to know that I'm not going to dispense any expert advice in response to her query, Jane advances a theory of her own.

> You know, for as long as I can remember I've been worried what other people think of me. I think I'm worried about being judged. Like if someone were to judge me in a way that made me feel bad, I just couldn't tolerate it. I get so worried about that it's like I lose my own humanness. I feel as though I have to put up this huge wall or something to keep myself safe.

I pause for a few beats to let Jane feel the profundity of her own words.

> Jane, is it your belief that something has happened in the last little while that has started to tear down that wall of judgment and anxiety?

An air of excitement starts to gain some momentum in Jane's being.

> This last week has been so crazy I don't even know if you would believe it. So, there's this woman who lives down the street from me. She had all of these

'Vote for Hillary' signs in her yard and stuff. Every day I would drive by them for like the last two years and just notice myself scowling. I don't know if she knows that I voted for Trump or not because I don't have signs or bumper stickers or any of that. Anyway, I drove by earlier this week and noticed that same scowl coming on. Then I had this like rush of panic. I was like, oh my god, this is exactly what I've been talking about with Travis! Here was a woman that I automatically thought I didn't like and never really gave her a chance. I tried to find ways to talk myself out of going to talk to her, but then I thought to myself, what would this humanness we've been talking about make me do?

Jane pauses for a few seconds, and I feel like an eager reader who can no longer contain himself from discovering what is on the next page.

"Well?!?" I exclaim, noticing my backside making its way to the edge of the chair.
What sort of counsel did humanness give you?
I want you to know I tried to avoid it, like I said. But I figured this is why I'm here, right? If I'm not going to give it a try what's the point of doing this with you, you know? The next evening, I was walking my dog and she was outside taking the trash out. I just gave her a friendly wave. She made a comment about how beautiful our dog was. I started asking her some questions about her landscaping, which I really do love. One thing leads to another and there we are talking for like an hour. My husband actually called me to make sure I was okay. And that's not even the crazy part! She invited me over for dinner last weekend.

Jane appears to be equal parts electrified and flummoxed. I inquire:

Is it alright if I ask you how dinner went, Jane?
Oh, it was really, really good. I noticed a lot of anxiety before it, but once I got over there and we started talking again everything settled down.
Do you mind if I ask if the topic of Trump or Hillary came up?

I ask this question with a little bit of hesitation but also a sense that I owe it to our work to broach it.

No, it never did. It's not like I was avoiding it or something. It's just that there were more interesting things to talk about.

The wall of judgment and politics would try and convince you that these differences must define the conversation, but somehow humanness helped you find a different direction?

Yeah, I guess that's right. It turns out that we actually have a lot in common. We both have adult sons. We both like to garden. We both have the same taste in music. And my husband and her husband really get along, too. I was almost a little embarrassed that it took me this long to get to know her.

What was it about the process of getting to know her that has helped erase anxiety in your life for the time being, Jane?

Jane leans back on the couch in deep contemplation, almost like she is studying the interactions with her neighbor for a clue that might help solve this mystery.

I don't know. If she can like me, maybe I'm not that bad? Maybe I don't have so much to worry about when I talk to other people? Of course, who knows what she would think if she knew that I voted for...you know, Trump.

A cold silence settles over our conversation. I can feel hope starting to slip out of our collective grasp.

Jane, do you mind if I ask your neighbor's name?

Deborah.

Jane, do you think this newly forming friendship you are creating with Deborah could withstand the realization that the two of you voted for different people?

Are you saying I should tell her?

I feel a little extra sting in Jane's words.

I remain silent with hopes that Jane takes some time to further evaluate this prospect.

Jane continues:

I mean, what if she gets angry or won't talk to me anymore?

This certainly comes with risk, doesn't it?

Jane nods.

> Can this humanness the two of you have created together get you through this challenge much the same way it helped us get through?
>
> Maybe, but she's not a therapist. What if it goes totally differently? What if she isn't as nice to me as you were?

Jane bounces her right leg nervously, the muscles in her face strain.

> Do you have some sense that because I'm a therapist I might have gone easy on you with regard to trying to reconcile our politics?

Jane pauses. The pressure in the room is now bearing down on my head, much the way it feels during an ascent to 30,000 feet in an airplane.

> "It's not like I think you were lying or something," Jane asserts, "but it is your job to be nice to me, right?"
>
> Is that my job?

I reply quickly. I feel like a shortstop that just made a throw and now wishes he could have it back moments after it leaves his fingertips.

> I guess not.

Jane's tone is sullen.
I gather myself.

> Jane, what might be the consequences of me being nice to you just for the sake of being nice? Would that be respectful of the work we are trying to do together?
>
> Yeah, I get what you're saying.

We leave the meeting both cloaked in uncertainty and unease. As I begin packing up my bag in preparation to leave the office, I worry that my invitation for Jane to broach the subject of politics with her neighbor and newfound friend may have pushed her too far. Did she take it as a mandate? Did I miscalculate our relationship and the trust I thought we had built together? Hell, maybe she was right, and I was just trying to be nice. This dubiety was hot on my tail between our meetings. A part of me wondered if she would even show up.

Two weeks later I find myself in the bathroom near my office looking in the mirror and feeling an air of anxiety I rarely feel, wondering how the conversation with Jane might take shape. I fretfully rub my chin, take a deep breath, and walk down to meet Jane. Our greeting seems unremarkable. As we walk towards the office, I pay close attention looking for some kind of sign to inform me how Jane might be feeling. I can find none.

As we sit down, I brace myself for what is to come. She begins the conversation with no prompting from me.

> I just want to say thank you.

I feel as disoriented, as I do astonished, by her opening statement.

> What?

This one-word question was all I could seem to muster in response.

> You pushed me to try and talk to Deborah about our politics, and you know, it was the right move.

I'm fixated on her use of the word "push," fearing that it might confirm one of my worst fears.

> Yeah, you know, Jane, I've been thinking a lot the past couple of weeks. I've wondered if perhaps I pushed too hard? In fact, I wish I would have done more inviting than pushing.
>
> Oh, I don't mean to say that I felt pushed like against my will or something like that. What I mean is that you helped me push through a hurdle I might not have pushed through by myself. It's almost like the way a personal trainer would help someone run a little harder than they might want to, you know?

I feel a bit of relief, but the tension doesn't exit my body completely.

> Jane, you said talking to Deborah about politics was the right move for you. Might I ask how you've come to understand that as true?

Jane chuckles warmly and, as she does, we reclaim some of our therapeutic rhythm.

> You're never going to believe this! When I brought up the idea of politics, she said she already knew I voted for Trump. I said to her that I didn't know it was that obvious.

I return the warm chuckle.

> That conversation sounds familiar, huh?

We both take a moment to reflect.

> Do you mind if I ask what happened next, Jane?
> Oh, well, it really wasn't too big of a deal. You know, I just made some joke about how we probably shouldn't like one another. We both laughed. Then we just kind of carried on as usual.

Committed to understanding this in more depth because of a deep sentiment that there might be value in doing so, I continue walking down this path with Jane.

> What do you think you gained by broaching this subject with Deborah as opposed to just ignoring it?
> It's like the big pink elephant in the room or whatever. We both knew it was there.
> Why not talk about it?
> It didn't come without risk, though, like you mentioned in our last meeting, right? What if it had gone poorly?
> Of course. But then we would have been building kind of a fake relationship, anyway.
> What about this conversation you had with Deborah made the relationship feel more real?

Jane's body leans into the conversation a little bit more.

> It boils down to can you like me, who I actually am? I've always felt that I had to be this specific person for everyone else. Basically, like the perfect person for them.

> Did it feel as though you had to be many different perfect people depending on who you were interacting with?

Jane's energy is now indisputable.

> Yes! I've been trying to be so many different people. After this conversation it's like I could just be one version of me.
>
> And would you say that this is the version of you that you like most?

I could sense a large lump forming in Jane's throat. A yelp launches from her mouth. She buries her head in her open palms and begins to weep. She begins talking with tears still cascading down her face.

> It's like I could never really be this person. I was trying to be someone for my dad. Then I was trying to be someone for my friends and my husband. Then when my kids were young, I was trying to be the right mom. I never felt like it was right to just be me. No one would really like me. Here's the thing, I think you really do like me even though we have these differences. You weren't just trying to be nice. I feel the same way about Deborah. If you and Deborah can both like me even though we have some major differences, maybe I can just be me. I can stop trying to be someone different for everyone. And that's such a huge relief. Do you know how exhausting that is?
>
> When you are just being you, what do you notice happens to the anxiety that brought you to see me?
>
> This is why I think it's gone. I mean, everyone has anxiety and stuff. It's not like I never feel it, but that big anxiety that landed me in the hospital is gone.

I pause for a few seconds sensing that we might be stumbling on something of paramount importance.

> Jane, I want to make sure I'm not getting this wrong. Are you saying that when you can be the most preferred version of yourself that anxiety from the past melts away?

She looks me in the eyes and says conclusively:

> Exactly.

> Do you think we could have discovered this if you and I had the same political beliefs or we didn't have the conversation about politics that we had a few weeks back?

Jane says firmly:

> I really don't think so. I thought I was going to come here to see you for anxiety and you were going to give me some techniques or something to fix it. I didn't think that who we are as people would even matter. I mean, I had never done anything like this. But this is so much deeper. To know that you actually like me despite that we voted for different people helped me learn something I didn't even know I needed to learn.
>
> Jane, do you think these ideas we've discovered in here are better than ideas we might have found in a book or on Google?

The corners of Jane's mouth turn upwards exposing a toothy grin.

> So much better.
>
> Might I ask why you experience it as better?
>
> Because we made this together. It just sort of happened. It didn't feel forced. It's like we just knew where to go, and even when we didn't, I always knew we would figure it out.

A coy grin slowly paints itself on my lips.

> Have you ever noticed that sometimes magic turns up in peculiar places, Jane?

She pauses to contemplate. The way her eyes start to dance let me know something is afoot.

> That's so funny you bring up magic. You know, my grandmother used to read me stories by Roald Dahl when I was a kid. Then she gave me this book by him called *The Minpins* shortly before she died when my kids were really little. I used to read this book to my kids every night when they got a little older. There is this line at the very end that goes, 'Those who don't believe in magic will never find it.' It's funny you bring up magic because I've always believed in magic. My husband actually still teases me about it to this day.

Jane's words leave me feeling an extra boost of therapeutic vitality.

> This is a major guess on my part, so I know I very well could be wrong here, Jane. But do you think we might have located some kind of most unlikely magic in here?

Jane takes some time to metabolize my question more fully.

> Well, I figured you'd done this sort of thing with other people like me before. Maybe not exactly the same, but you know, like pretty close.
>
> Can I tell you a dirty little secret, Jane? I've never done this kind of work we've done together with anyone before. And, to be honest, I'm quite certain I couldn't have pulled it off without you as my fellow trailblazer.

Jane gives a quick nod of appreciation.

> Jane, if you found out that I had performed this exact script with someone else might it have taken away from the magic?

She wastes no time in responding.

> Then it wouldn't be magical. I went to this other therapist some years ago, and I felt like he was doing what you just said with the script. It's like he had done this a thousand times before and was just cashing checks. I've always felt like you really care, like beyond just making money. You ask these questions that you could only ask by listening very carefully to me, and I don't just mean the words that come out of my mouth. You listen deeper than that. And you ask questions that I just can't shake. It's like you think about every word that comes out of your mouth. You are so careful to try and get every word right. It doesn't mean they are easy questions or that they always feel good, but I told my husband the other night there's at least one question you ask each time that follows me wherever I go. I can't get it out of my head.
>
> If you were to summarize what it is about this work we've done as a whole that will stick with you and that you might not be able to get out of your head or your heart, what might that summary include?
>
> If someone that is supposed to hate me can invest this much in me, maybe I'm not such a bad person. Maybe I'm okay. Maybe we are okay?
>
> Maybe we *are* okay.

Jane and I smile at one another in solidarity, the kind that not even political vitriol could divide.

After this meeting comes to a close, we have a couple of more conversations per her request to make sure the new relationship she is forming with anxiety has some staying power. I hear from Jane every so often via phone or text with small updates about her life. Over three years later, she still reflects on our work together as something that is of value for her. As valuable as it has been for her, I often wonder if it has been of even more value for me.

My conversations with Jane are leading me to question what it means to be a therapist motivated by "social justice." These conversations have also prompted me to consider looking for a new term altogether. This original idea of justice work in in psychotherapy is supposed to be radical, but I wonder if it is being enacted in a way that can sometimes invite therapists to consider that they can only work with people who have the same core beliefs and ways of living as them. Jane has invited me to consider, what is more radical than working with someone who society forbids you from being relationally connected to? If I am deterred from seeing people with different political beliefs than me, in what ways am I replicating the same national trauma that's taking place daily in United States?

Since our formal meetings together have come to an end, Jane has sent a number of people my way to engage in conversations. One such woman makes her way to my office and says something I won't soon forget.

> I hear you're the therapist who will work with anyone, even us deplorables who voted for Trump.

I respond with a coy grin.

> Without difference, is there any hope for progress?

And just like that, I feel us being pulled away again in the river of paradox left only to trust where its currents might take us.

Section III

A Teaching Story

Given that this book shares both practical and pedagogical purposes, this next chapter introduces readers to an example of our pedagogy through a teaching story. In this story, Travis Heath takes readers through a workshop with participants using his practice story, ""*Maybe We Are Okay:*" Contemporary Narrative Therapy in the Time of Trump."

The hope of this teaching story is to take readers inside our proposed pedagogy through a dialogue between teacher and workshop participants.

Imagine for a moment that you have signed up for a two-day narrative therapy workshop. You feel a wave of excitement as you think about attending alongside a group of people who share your passion for reimagining all that a therapeutic conversation could be. You pull out your phone and peruse the brochure one last time. The thought of moving away from therapy manuals that have become stale for you is intriguing but also a bit scary. Questions start running laps in your mind. How will this actually work? Will I be able to do it? How exactly is this guy going to use stories to teach therapy, anyway? As you walk closer to the door of the classroom, you push pause on the doubt and lean into a sense of wonder and curiosity. You take one last deep breath and enter the room. The journey begins...

DOI: 10.4324/9781003226543-10

CHAPTER 8

INSPIRITED CONTEMPORARY NARRATIVE THERAPY
A Two-Day Workshop

TRAVIS HEATH

I am always nervous speaking with a group of people I have never met before. Today is no exception. I have arrived ahead of time in a classroom that can accommodate 30 or more.

I hook-up my computer to the projector to test it out. I make small talk to those nearby in an attempt to settle my nerves. The clock strikes 10 am. All the seats are occupied with a few people standing in the back of the room and the staff rushing to find some extra chairs.

I inhale deeply before beginning.

> Hello everyone. I want you to know how much it means to me that all of you would sign-up to spend the next two days together. It just really means a lot to me. Thank you.

I see a few faces flash friendly smiles in response to my introduction. This helps me settle in somewhat.

> I was wondering if I might start by just asking about the level of familiarity with narrative therapy for everyone in the room. May I ask how many of you were aware of narrative therapy prior to coming to this workshop?

Most of the people in the room raise their hands. A woman named Bella, a licensed counselor for a decade who is new to narrative therapy, adds:

> Well, familiar, yeah. But I wouldn't say I know that much about it. That's why I'm here.

A few of the other attendees nod as if to indicate they are in the same boat.

> Okay, thank you for that. Are there any folks who would say they have a long history with narrative therapy, maybe even practice it in their work?

Five people raise their hands.

> How about people who are brand new to narrative work? Would you mind raising your hands?

Eight brave souls indicate that this was completely new terrain for them.

> I just want to say that all of you are welcome here. My hope is that regardless of your history with narrative ideas and practice that our time together might invite you into *feeling* the work in ways that might be interesting and hopefully useful to each and every one of you.

The room generally feels warm and receptive. I'm already feeling a connection to the people with whom I'm sharing the space.

> I'm wondering if we might start this off a little differently than many of you are likely accustomed to. How many of you when you learn about a way of practicing therapy start with theory, often PowerPoints about theory?

The group gives a sort of unanimous groan.

> Oh, is it fair to say that PowerPoints aren't your favorite?

Jerry, a longtime therapist, in the first row perks up and says:

> To be honest, that's one of the big reasons I came here. I heard you don't use PowerPoints in these workshops.

That's music to my ears, brother. Okay, here's my proposal, and it's one that might seem a little bit backwards by traditional standards. I have a story I'd like to share with you. It's not just a transcript; it's actually a story. I hope this story can take you inside one of the conversations I was having with a woman named Jane. If the story is doing the work that I hope it will, it will reveal what I am going to refer to as the 'spirits' of this conversation. And my intention is that we might just focus on the story itself and not worry about connecting it to any kind of theory at first. Is what I'm saying making sense so far?

They nod affirmatively.

Great. I'm glad to know we're on the same page so far. If it's alright with all of you, I'll put the story on the big screen so that you can read it as we go along. At any time, please feel free to stop me if you have a question or comment about anything. As well, I might stop and pose some questions to the group as well. Does this sound okay? For those of you familiar with conventional therapeutic practice, can we avoid using typical therapeutic or even narrative therapy lingo?

The group looks a bit off kilter for the first time. This excites me.
A woman named Helen, a newly minted psychologist sitting in the first row, asks:

You mean like not calling something 'externalization?'

Precisely! For those of you who may not know, externalization is among the most popular of narrative terms. Instead of using this kind of already popularized language, might we come up with our own language and vocabularies to describe what we are seeing and feeling?

A young woman near the back of the room hesitantly raises her hand.

But I'm a graduate student, and I don't even know that much about narrative therapy. So, I'm thinking this could be really hard for people in my position.

Do you mind if I ask your name?

Sure. It's Jessica.

I really want to thank you for your comment, Jessica. I'm wondering as we progress through the story, and we see certain practices, if we might

207

stop, see what's kicking around in our bodies, minds, hearts, and souls, and then find appropriate vocabulary. It doesn't have to be professionalized language. In fact, I wonder if there might be some benefit to it not being professionalized? When I've taught like this before I've noticed that people often feel like they won't be able to do it initially, but once they get in the groove, they discover they might be a bit better at it than they anticipated.

Jessica smiles warmly, seemingly comforted by my proposal.

> I have just one more overture I'd like to make. I wonder as we go through the story if you might begin to pay attention to the guiding narrative 'spirits' of my work?

I pause purposefully, expecting that the word 'spirits' might lead to some discomfiture. It's apparent after just a few seconds that this is the case, judging by the looks on the faces of several people.
Jerry replies:

> Well, what do you mean when you say 'spirits' of practice? I've never heard that term before.
> Yes, it's not the kind of term we often hear in our formal training programs, is it?
> I'm wondering, Jerry, if you or anyone else could muster a guess as to what we might be getting at with this term narrative 'spirits' of practice.

There is an uncomfortable silence. I notice a twinkle in Jessica's eyes that seems to be wrestling with uncertainty. She proposes:

> Uh, this might not be right, but...umm...maybe by spirits you mean like what's at the core of your work?
> Ooh, I really like the word you chose there, Jessica, *core*. This immediately has me thinking about a fruit, for example. Without its core, can a fruit survive? Would it be fair to say the core gives life to rest of the fruit, and without it, the fruit could not survive? What might be at the core of our practices that gives life to the sweet and edible exterior? And without a strong core, might the exterior rot?

I pause momentarily and try to take the pulse of the room. There seems to be a bit of angst swimming around, but the good kind.

> Is this idea of 'spirits' as being at the core of our practices resonating with anyone else?

Some people tentatively and perhaps grudgingly nod in the affirmative, and Helen says:

> I think of the words 'ethics' or 'values.'.
> This is a keen observation, Helen. In fact, my colleagues and I used to use both of these words frequently. Not that long ago we made the shift to 'spirits' Do you have any sense why we might have made that shift? Do you think the word 'spirits' might offer anything distinctive from the words ethics and values?

Maya, a senior woman near the back of the room raises her hand and stands to speak.

> Well, I'm 67 years old, so maybe I think about this idea of therapy a little differently than I'm supposed to, but when I hear the word 'spirits,' I think of something more mystical. It reminds me of going to church with my grandmother in Alabama when I was a young girl. I can feel that word in my body. When I hear 'ethics' and 'values', I don't feel anything.

I find myself moving closer to her with each word she utters as though I was under her spell.

> I think you've captured it in a way I haven't been able to, Maya. What might be the consequences of our practices appealing only to the brains and minds of people and not to their hearts and souls? Might we put the story of Jane consulting with me and go through it together and as we do, we can begin to identify the 'spirits' of practice that were guiding our work?

Jessica raises her hand with a look of consternation.

> But some of us are just meeting you for the first time. How would we know what your 'spirits' are?

209

> Oh, Jessica! My hope is that the questions you will soon read are more than just an intellectual exercise, but rather, constructed in such a way that they have heart and soul that one can feel. Now, perhaps not every question will meet this ideal, but I'm hoping there might be at least a few. If so, might we take a shot at creating a vocabulary for the 'spirits' you feel in my questions?

An apprehensive and curious energy passes through the room.

> Here's the thing; it would be really hard to be wrong because surely there are 'spirits' guiding my work of which I'm not even aware. Or perhaps you might have a way of describing the 'spirits' you perceive better than any vocabulary I've created or adopted to date. I think we would agree that there are some questions that are surely not narrative in spirit, maybe the kind you would find, for example, in a standard psychiatric interview. Would you be willing to join me in this venture over the next couple of days?

The group consents despite a growing uncertainty about what is to come next. I open Jane's story on my computer and project it on the big screen. Just before I'm set to begin, Helen speaks politely:

> Travis, I have just one more thing I'm wondering about. You mentioned our theories of change. What about what our clients think about change?

I can hardly contain my enthusiasm.

> Wow, what great questions this groups asks! What if I proposed to the group that one of my 'spirits' of narrative practice is to elevate the knowledge of the person I'm speaking with? I might call this a spirit of dignification that has me try and honor the person I'm speaking with and their knowledges and understandings of the world. Do you think we can see how successful I was in bringing a spirit of dignification to the conversation with Jane. And if I was successfully able to turn this spirit into practice?
> On the dry erase board, I write the phrase, "Spirits of Narrative Practice" and jot down "Dignification" underneath it.
> Do you think we might keep a list of the 'spirits' of narrative practice that are showing up in the conversation with Jane and try and pay close attention to how they are manifesting in the questions?

This example seems to offer the group more clarity that it had perhaps been craving.

> Again, can I invite us to try and stay away from professional languages. Maybe we can do what Maya suggested earlier and see what words the feelings in our bodies invite us into using? Also, as I start reading the story, please stop me at any point with questions, concerns, critiques, and so on.

I begin reading Jane's story, matching what I am reading with the text on the screen. I take care to ensure that I am performing the words rather than just reading. My attempts to have them 'feel', and not just 'hear', appear to be successful as I notice the group beginning to lean forward in unison just a couple of minutes into the storytelling.

As I read the passage in which Jane and I have a conversation about who we voted for in the 2016 Presidential election, the room begins to stir. I make the calculation to pause for the first time.

> I'm just guessing, and I know I could be wrong, but did some of you have a reaction to that last exchange between Jane and me?

A collective giggle overtakes the room, confirming my suspicion. A prolonged silence follows. Finally, Jerry chimes in.

> Well, I think the interesting thing is you engaged in self-disclosure that you're usually taught not to do. We could also see what was going on in your head, your internal deliberations. I've never really seen that before.

We go back to that specific part of the text and I read it aloud again beginning with Jane's question:

> *'You voted for Hillary, didn't you?'*
>
> *The question doesn't quite feel accusatory, but the words travel crisply enough through the air to stir up a bit of tension.*
>
> *My mind is racing trying to prepare a suitable response. I can hear in my mind's ear the professors who administered much of my formal training prohibiting any self-disclosure and instead advising responses of this sort, 'That's an interesting question. I wonder what makes you ask that?' I shake off such a suggestion and almost chuckle out loud knowing that she knows me well enough at this stage to call bullshit on such a charade.*

211

> *I pause, consulting other mentors and prized elders who have helped me along my path to becoming a therapist. I know what I have to do.*
>
> *'Yeah, I did,' I respond endeavoring to strike a tone of openness blended with steadfastness.*

I re-engage the group.

> Jerry, you brought up the idea of self-disclosure. Did you hear this mentioned a lot in your training as I did?

A raucous reaction breaks out with laughter and chatter among participants, clearly in agreement with my observation. Jerry continues:

> Yeah, it was always something that I was taught to be very cautious about. In fact, some of my professors basically said you should avoid it all together. It just seemed like a risky move there to disclose whom you voted for.

I pause and rub my chin.

> I have a question that has surfaced in my mind. I don't know if it will prove to be helpful. What's the difference between self-disclosing and being a person?

The silence that follows is in stark contrast to the rowdy laughter that ensued moments before.
Bella chimes in.

> Well, I guess self-disclosure is specific to being a therapist.

I pose another question to the group.

> Have you found this term self-disclosure to be helpful to the work you do with people who consult you or not so helpful?

After taking some time to think, Jessica advances an answer.

> I know I'm not supposed to say this, but I don't think it's been very helpful. It makes me feel paralyzed sometimes. I don't know who I'm supposed to be in the room.

> Perhaps I might be breaking a traditional rule of psychotherapy here, huh? What might be the cost to the person I'm in conversation with, if I fail to be a person? Would I be rendered a therapy-bot of some kind, that artificial intelligence could replace?

Warm laughter cascades through the room.

> I want to be clear that it's not like I spend most of the meeting talking about me, but do I perhaps owe it to the people who seek my counsel to be fully me? Or least the best understanding of me I currently have? By the way, do you suppose we might be stumbling upon a spirit of practice here? If so, what might we call it?

The group assumes a pensive demeanor, followed by a protracted silence. I make the calculated choice to let the silence continue as long as is needed, knowing that the capacity to engage around questions like this one will be fundamental to the overall success of the workshop.
Helen breaks the silence.

> Maybe... authenticity?

I see an opportunity to be intentional about our use of language.

> Thanks for this, Helen. I think the word authenticity, in terms of its literal definition, fits really nicely here. I wonder, though, if it is a word that has been so professionalized that it has perhaps lost its originality. What do you think? Have you heard this before in your training?

The group nods in unison.

> Is there perhaps a different way we could express this that might breathe some life into it?

I see a bevy of furrowed brows deep in contemplation staring back at me. As I scan the room, I notice a flicker of electricity in Maya's eyes and feel a sense of anticipation that she might be preparing to offer us more of her wisdom.

> The word that comes to mind for me is 'wholehearted.'

There is a purr of agreement in response from the group. I grab the marker and add 'wholehearted' to our list.

> Do you think sometimes therapy training as usual mandates that we be half-hearted therapists? What might be the consequences of such a practice?

Maya continues.

> They don't really know *you* if only some of your heart is allowed in.
> And what is the potential of having two whole hearts creating something together? Could the results be exponential? Maybe we can continue to look for a spirit of wholeheartedness and see if this was implicated in any questions that I asked Jane?
> The group concurs. I notice we are already 90 minutes into our work together and propose that we take a short break. I slip out the back door of the classroom and go for a quick walk. I play back certain moments in my mind. Jessica's willingness to speak, given her neophyte status, makes me smile. Maya's ancestral wisdom feels like something that will likely come in handy throughout our two days together.

On my return, I begin performing the story after the revelation of Jane and my voting preferences, reading the following passage:

> *"Wow!" I exclaim. "Don't you think this is amazing?"*
> *She cocks her head in utter confusion, seemingly baffled.*
> *"May I ask you a question?" I say with a bit of a twinkle in my eye. She nods her assent.*
> *Do you like me as a human being?*
> *"Of course I do," she replies without hesitation.*
> *"May I share something with you?" I continue. She gestures for me to continue with a quick nod of her head. "I like you, too."*

Jerry's hand shoots into the air.

> There's that wholehearted idea we were talking about again. Because you didn't just ask if she liked you, you also shared that you liked her. There's a reciprocity to it.

I reengage with the story. As it progresses, Jane and I find ourselves diving even deeper into our own personal political differences and the differences in our country. While seemingly enthralled with the story, there was also an unease that had found its way into the room. Heidi gave words to this sentiment.

> It feels like you are talking about something with Jane that you're not supposed to talk about. You didn't just admit that you voted for Hillary and she voted for Trump and move on. It's like you're going deeper into politics. You are holding your position, but also allowing her to hold hers.

Acknowledging the value of Heidi's observation, we continue on with the story. The inquiry into party politics continues and so too does the uncertainty of the group. I read aloud the following question I asked Jane:

> *Once you got here and we began our work together, what was it that made you trust I would take good care of your stories even despite the fact that we might have been placed by the world into two different political camps?*

A coy grin gradually takes over Jerry's face.

> Personally, I like how you talk about taking good care of her stories. That's just a really nice phrase. But what I was really struck by is how you described being placed by the world into different political parties.

He pauses to study the question.

> It's just we usually don't think about political parties as something we're placed into, especially not in this day and age. It's more of a choice we make. Can you talk about that?
>
> It's a really great question, Jerry, and I appreciate the careful attention to detail. I guess I just get really skeptical anytime I'm presented with a dichotomy. I hear a lot of, 'we've got to listen to both sides' these days. Every time I hear someone say this, it really bugs me because I feel like there are almost always more than two sides. Do we risk limiting people and relationships if we restrict ideas to only two sides of a single coin? And if we believe that there are usually more than two sides, then have we been in some way

215

forced into one of the two political parties in United States that may not truly represent the totality of our interests?

As the group is taking some time to let my response marinate, I see Jessica becoming somewhat uneasy. I provide a subtle and friendly nod to encourage her to speak. After a slight pause, she says:

> When you were describing this, I thought of a flower. Before a flower blooms, it is just a single bulb, but once it blooms there are many petals. That's kind of what this question felt like to me.

I walk toward the whiteboard.

> That's a lovely description, Jessica. Might we call it a 'flower' question?

She smiles.

> Yeah, I like that.

I reciprocate the smile.

> That's a little different than the kind of language we might typically use to describe therapy, huh?

The group collectively chuckles.

> You've got me thinking, Jessica. I think that flower questions might be seminal to my practice. For example, when someone I'm in conversation with says they are depressed, I often ask, what kind of depression is it? Is it one that serves them or doesn't serve them? Would they like to keep it around or not? Or maybe there are parts they would like to keep around and other parts they wouldn't? I think you get the idea. I guess my hope is that such a flower question takes it from a single bulb of depression to one that might bloom into many other petals of possibility and understanding.

Helen raises her hand and makes an observation:

> I notice that you talk about the questions that go through your head as you're thinking of them for us to see but don't necessarily share aloud with Jane. You've already done that quite a bit. Can you tell us why you do that?

> In all seriousness, I have to tell you, Helen, this is such a relief to hear you say this. Part of the reason we've tried to write this way is in hopes that we might get the very reaction you've had. Just watching a therapy session live or on video or to read a transcript doesn't really allow someone to figure out how the therapist made up his or her mind. I get credit for asking a certain question, but when you read what I was thinking that led to my question, you might discover that the person responding to the question has made much more of it than I could ever have imagined!

Feeling like the topic was sufficiently addressed, at least for now, we continue on with the story and arrive at a point in the conversation where Jane and I were exploring the taboo around politics and religion.

> *"I'm fairly certain my field abides by this idea that religion and politics are often subjects that should be for the most part avoided, too" I explain. "Why do you think it is that both of us chose to break this rule in our conversation tonight? Did you have any sense that there might be value in doing so?"*

I sense an opportunity to explore the work further.

> Is there any language that sticks out to you in those last couple of questions?
> Several shout-out "break this rule" in unison.
> What is it in particular about the idea of rule-breaking that seems to be doing something of possible importance here?

Jerry, the veteran narrative practitioner in the room, catches the question almost before it has time to leave my mouth.

> I first saw David and Michael give workshops about 25 years ago. It always struck me that they were breaking certain rules of therapy. I don't know if they ever came out and said it in quite the way you did, but I think it was implied. That's what made it so exciting to me.

Hoping Jerry might expand on this, I ask:

> Would you say that it's important to have rules in therapy?

Jerry takes this up.

Well, yeah. We obviously need some rules. But shouldn't we at least try and understand why we have the rules we do?

Are you by chance saying, Jerry, that some rules are kept with very little, if any, examination?

Jerry concludes:

Oh, absolutely!

I address the group.

Do you think the same rules should apply for every person we're in conversation with? What might be the consequences of such a policy?

Jessica accepts my invitation.

There should probably be basic rules. You know, like treat people with respect. After that, though...I don't know.

Do you suppose that breaking rules might have the ability to expand possibility?

I'm met with disquiet.

For example, if a person comes to therapy knowing, or strongly suspecting that topics like politics and religion are off the table to talk about in substantive and challenging ways, could that limit the possibilities for where our conversation might go? And if we were to at least explore putting these topics on the table, an exploration that the person we're speaking with has the unquestionable right to adjudicate, could we then find matters that otherwise couldn't be considered?

Jessica offers another reply.

My gut says, yes. I just also think there is risk involved.

I don't think there's any doubt that there's risk involved, Jessica. I suppose risk is scary because we can't know the outcome, wouldn't you say?

She nods in agreement.

> Could it also be simultaneously exciting in that it could open up unexplored terrain? And can we trust ourselves and the relationship we share with the people we are in conversation with to abandon this exploration if it becomes perilous?

Thinking it might be helpful to give the group an example of this practice, I read something I asked Jane a little further down the page.

> *As we are talking about it now are you finding it to be of any value or do you think it would serve us better to go in another direction?*
>
> *She thinks diligently about my query before reaching her solution. "Now that you mention it, I feel like we are being more real with each other. It's also like rebellious or something."*

I quickly attempt to tie this back to what we were just talking about hoping that it's applicability won't get lost.

> You know, if she had said this wasn't of value, I would have immediately asked her if she would prefer to exit this conversation. And to be honest, it would have been no skin off my back. I'm just not that interested in any proposal I make being the 'right' one. What I'm really interested in is discovering directions together that might prove helpful based on the person's knowledge of themselves and the world. Also, imagine my proposal offended her in some way. I actually look at this as an opportunity. It gives me a chance to apologise and seek repair, which I've come to learn any relationship is going to need to call upon at some point. Why would our relationship be any different?

Jerry flashes a friendly smile.

> See, there you go again?

I cock my head in curiosity.

> You're breaking rules again. Therapists are supposed to be petrified of offending their clients, like it's the worst thing you could do. But there you go talking about it in a different way as though it's normal or something.

I chuckle, reciprocating Jerry's playful tone.

> Do you think there might be a spirit of practice here in all of this?

Maya leans forward uttering just two words.

> Rebel love.

A collective gasp follows.

> Wow! What a phrase, Maya! I love it. I just hope I can do it some measure of justice.

I write it on our board.
I notice that another hour and a half has melted away.

> Ooh, I'm sorry. I know we've been going for a while. Maybe we should take a break for lunch now and return around 1:30?

As everyone reassembles, the decibel level doubles. I utter several friendly shouts prompting us to reengage with my performance of the text of the interview.

> "You know, just this idea that two people would be so different because of who they voted for," Jane asserts. "Maybe we're not that different. Or even if we are different in certain ways maybe that is only on the surface."
> Do you think it feels unfair that we have basically only been given two options?
> Without hesitating Jane emphatically replies, "Yes!"

Helen invites me to pause.

> Isn't that what we were calling a flower question earlier?
> How do you mean?
> Well, you asked is it unfair that you only get two options. That's the bulb blooming into the petals, right?

I pump my fist in excitement.

> I think she's spot-on. What do all of you think?

The group seems to share my excitement regarding this development.

> Hey, I know we haven't made it to the end of our first day together yet, but is it alright if I circle back to a conversation that we were having a bit earlier? Jessica, you voiced some concerns about trying to make sense of this idea of 'spirits of practice' and how it might play out in an actual conversation. I'm wondering, have we made any headway with that? Or, maybe I'm getting ahead of myself here.

Jessica is quick to respond, quite unlike the initial impression she gave of being a shy neophyte therapist.

> It's making a lot more sense, more sense than narrative therapy has made before. I can definitely see it now.

Not about to let me off the hook, she adds:

> I still don't know if I can do it on my own. I can see how you do it, which is really helpful though.
>
> You seem to have a penchant for reading my mind, Jessica, because my hope is that by the end of our time together tomorrow you can begin to identify some of your 'spirits of practice' and perhaps envision what questions they might encourage you to ask.

Returning to the story, we reach the final moments of the first conversation I had with Jane where we began looking at the petals of possibility the flower question had gifted us. Most specifically, the idea that we might be creating something that is neither Trump nor Hillary.

A conversation I had with myself, on the drive home, follows:

> *What will my narrative therapy friends think about this? Am I selling out by working with a Trump supporter? Am I practicing the wrong kind of 'social justice?'*
>
> I notice a look of consternation mixed with contemplation as I catch a quick glance of my face in the rearview mirror. I can feel rebuttals brewing in my soul.
>
> *What is social justice, anyway? Might I need to start anew and refashion my understanding of social justice? Have I been adhering to a canonized version of social justice that could engage in the same damaging habit that social justice movements had set out to try and avoid in the first place?*

A serious silence blankets the room. I decide to ask a question.

> Might I ask what my narrative therapy friends in the room today think about me working with a Trump supporter? Have I sold out? Have I betrayed social justice?

Bella, who hadn't yet said much so far, breaks the silence.

> A big part of why I have started reading a little about narrative therapy is because of the social justice component. My friend, who had been to one of your workshops last year, said that she loved your commitment to social justice.

Bella's voice trails off, and I wonder if she is now questioning my commitment to the very idea that encouraged her to come to this workshop in the first place. Perhaps some of my concerns about sharing this part of my conversation with Jane are coming to life in real time. I push through the tension.

> Do you ever notice that a phrase sometimes starts to lose its meaning? For example, I hear the term multicultural counseling all the time now. It seems every psychology, counseling, social work program uses this phrase. It's become a box to check. At one time, I imagine that the notion of multicultural counseling was quite provocative. I wonder now if that time has passed. Does language have a shelf life? If that is so, do we have to come up with new language? This is something that some of my colleagues and I have started doing with the phrase 'anti-colonial counseling' or the term 'cultural democracy' as possible alternatives. As this portion of the story reveals, I have been having the same reservations around the term social justice for a few years now. If everyone is practicing social justice, is anyone *really* practicing it? Moreover, if I refuse to work with a person based on their political beliefs, where exactly is the justice in that?

It's almost as though the tension I felt in the conversation with Jane has leapt off the screen and is permeating the workshop. While uncomfortable, perhaps the story is doing the work it was designed to do in this moment.

> I must admit that I wrote this story largely in an attempt to try and explain to myself what was happening in my conversation with Jane. Many colleagues

tell me they could never work with a Trump supporter. That always felt uncomfortable to me. The challenge was that I didn't necessarily know quite how I would go about having such a conversation, only that I felt it unethical to avoid it outright. Might I pose the same question I did just a couple of minutes ago? Do you believe that I may have betrayed social justice by having this conversation with Jane?

So much time elapsed that I wondered if I should break the silence. Bella comes to our rescue.

> If I'm being honest, I did wonder if you were 'betraying social justice' when you first read that part from the story. After listening to you speak about it for a little bit though, it's got me thinking that maybe social justice has become a little limiting in certain ways. And you know, I'm conflicted because I've said before that I don't think I could work with Trump supporters.

A few of the other participants nod in agreement with Bella's sentiments. Helen adds:

> Yeah, I'm feeling the same way. If I was to say I was open to working with a Trump supporter, I might be endorsing some of what Trump stands for.

Helen also seems to be speaking to something others in attendance can identify with. I take a break from the palpable angst to admire what the story has stirred up.

> Look, I want you to know how much I appreciate what Bella and Helen have shared. May I admit that I've had many of the same thoughts? That's why I found it so important to take on the challenge of working with someone who had very different political beliefs from me. I entered this process not knowing exactly how to go about it, and as you can see by the progression of the story, it has kind of sneaked up on both of us after the election. It's certainly an imperfect dance Jane and I are in together.

Helen asks with spirited curiosity:

> How did you do it if you didn't know how you were going to do it before seeing Jane?

223

I pause and grin out of respect for the forthrightness of Helen's inquiry.

> I guess the best way I can answer this, Helen, is to say that I can't always make sense of what I'm doing it until I go back after the fact and look. These kinds of stories actually prove really helpful with this. Upon further review, what I'd like to say is that I was practicing with Jane something that Art Frank and Sylvia Naiden call 'radical respect.' I've heard Art say that he believes this is at the heart of narrative therapy (private correspondence, 2019). Is there a way for me to practice respect in our conversation that Jane can't help but feel even in spite our differences? And if I'm going to do this even somewhat successfully, might it be imperative that I interrogate the ideas that I hold close?

> I grab the marker and write the term "radical respect" on the board.

> Is it alright if I keep going with the story here? I wonder if perhaps we might seem to have as the conversation proceeds, an example of, or at least an attempt at, 'radical respect?'

I then asked Jane:

> What *bits of humanity am I getting to see in you that I might otherwise have missed out on had I not broken ranks with my group?*

I pose a question to the attendees.

> Can anyone, by chance, see a spirit of radical respect in this question?

The group takes a moment to ponder my query. Maya breaks the silence.

> The act of, as you say, breaking ranks with your group, is a radical act. Therapists aren't typically required to do this. And even if they do, they certainly aren't required to share it. I think to do so is a respectful act, but outside the way you would usually think, you know, by practicing empathy or something of that nature.

I take up where she left off.

> If I am willing to risk operating outside of my position, do you think that might invite Jane to do the same? And hey, it's not like we can't reassume the positions we came in with, right? They will still be there waiting for us.

I continue reading the story, inviting us to pay close attention to how Jane responds to my attempts at a question of 'radical respect' and what someone with different political beliefs might learn about her as a result.

> *Jane's tone feels more vulnerable as she responds, "That I'm a caring person. That I will go to the ends of the earth for the people I love." Jane pauses and begins to cry. "That I love all of God's creatures, even those different from me."*
>
> *Jane begins to sob more intensely and places her face in her palms. She then waves her left hand quickly as if to try and shake off the tears. "My dad was a Republican," she declares. "After he died, I felt a kind of responsibility to carry this on. Not that I do it just for him, but I know it was important to him. I know he wouldn't be pleased with everything about Trump. But I was forced into picking him, you know! I mean, what were my other options? I don't want to let my dad down. It's not like Trump was all bad or something, but I just felt trapped by the whole thing."*

Tears well up in the eyes of some of the participants, and I feel a lump in my throat. I slowly sit down in a chair, assuming an uncharacteristic stillness.

> Is it alright if I inquire what might be driving some of the tears that have found us in this room in this moment?

A protracted silence follows which persists. Bella clears her throat and takes what I suspect is a considerable risk.

> It's like I see Jane in a new light or something now. I am someone who really doesn't like Trump, but I am guilty of grouping all, or most all, Trump supporters together. When she started talking about her relationship with her father....

Bella's voice trails off and she begins to tear up but regains her composure.

> My father died two years ago. When she was talking about her father's legacy, something just really rang true for me.

I try to hold the endowment Bella handed over to us with appropriate reverence.

> I wonder, when we hear about many instances, does it become almost too abstract for us to really care? Is the term 'Trump supporters' so broad that

it's hard to find the humanity in that? Does paying close attention to the particular, and the unique, move us in ways adhering to the general cannot?

The group murmurs their agreement. I gently tug on the thread of "radical respect" just a little harder in continuing the story.

> *Might I apologize, Jane, for having prejudged you based on who you voted for?*
>
> *"What do you mean?" Jane replies, her eyes straining with perplexity.*
>
> *Is it possible I might have insulted a part of you that is deeply connected to your family and whom you know yourself to be?*
>
> *Jane shakes her head from left to right in a determined fashion and declares, "No, I never felt insulted by you."*

The group leans forward, almost as if being pulled by a magnet. My voice remains tender.

> It's reasonable to suggest that I could have gone in any number of directions here and, as is often the case, many of those directions could have been fruitful. Is the direction I chose one that might in any way live up to what we've cited as 'radical respect?'

Bella, doubtlessly still feeling the presence of her father as a companion in our conversation, is quick to take up my question.

> You are showing respect for her father and her family even though her father may have held political beliefs opposite from your own.

This response seems to ignite something in the rest of the group as hands shoot skyward. Helen adds:

> I might not be right here, but it's almost like you are apologizing for more than just you. Maybe she could start to feel like if you can see this and apologize, others might too if they knew her in the same way are starting to know her.

Jerry replies, almost snatching Helen's words in mid-flight:

> Yeah, if you can admit that you might have prejudged her, and you still like her as you established in the first meeting, maybe this can be done with others in her world, too.

A tinge of excitement starts to pulsate in the room. I slowly stand-up as I start to feel the energy shifting in my body.

> Hey, did y'all read ahead in the story?

The group flashes a look of confusion.

> I just ask because I think what you're saying is foreshadowing the very place I'm hoping to go.

I offer a coy grin that leads to chuckling from the attendees.
I glance at the clock in the back of the room and notice that the end of our time together is growing nigh.

> Geez, we only have about 10 minutes left for today. It feels like time is just running away from us. I usually find that is a good sign for how things are going along, but I feel like I could go another few hours. Don't worry, I won't subject you to such torture.

The attendees grant me a courtesy laugh in recognition of my feeble attempt at humor so late in the day.

> Are there any lingering questions or loose ends that I might help tie up before we part for the day?

Jerry tentatively raises his hand.

> I don't want to open up a can of worms or anything....

I smile and say warmly:

> I prefer eating my worms late in the afternoon. Go right ahead, Jerry.

Jerry reciprocates my playful tone:

> Well, in that case... in all seriousness, I've heard the idea that narrative therapists should be decentered. There's also this idea of being decentered but influential. Where do you stand on that?

As this is not the first time that I've heard someone bring up this topic during a workshop of mine, I have an inkling from past interactions as to what Jerry may be getting at.

> I don't in any way want to put words in your mouth here, Jerry, so tell me if I've got this wrong. I'm wondering if you might be experiencing me as not decentered enough?

He is measured in the tone of his reply.

> I actually like it, to be honest. But I just wonder if this is different than how some people have done narrative therapy.

Sensing this might be an opportunity to highlight an important idea in the practice of Contemporary Narrative Therapy, I am eager to extend the conversation.

> Might I ask what you notice about what I'm doing that feels different? And don't worry about saying something critical, Jerry. I'm not easily offended.

Jerry accepts my invitation.

> Again, I don't think it's a bad thing, but I notice that you are adding some of your own words. The way I was taught narrative therapy is that you should only use the words of the client.

I nod knowingly at Jerry's observation.

> I'm really glad you brought this up. I think it's an observation that some classical narrative therapists make quite frequently of my practice. First, if you were to read a letter that I write to the people who consult me, you would likely notice that it is composed largely of words that came out of their mouths. It's not that I don't believe in using that language. In fact, I find it to be very important. I guess I'm also interested in how such language came to be. Sometimes it might be language the person was already carrying with them prior to our conversation. Other times, that language might have come about as a result of our conversation. In other words, the questions I ask might have helped introduce language that otherwise wouldn't have

emerged. David Epston often cites the words of Ludwig Wittgenstein, *'The limits of my language are the limits of my mind. All I know is what I have words for.'*[1] What might be the consequences if I don't introduce new language? Are the people who are consulting me then confined to the very worlds in which they often feel so trapped to begin with?

Even despite the long day we have spent together, I make a quick scan of the room and see the group still apparently engaged. I make eye-contact with Jerry to offer him a chance to give his thoughts in case what I had said was in some way unclear.

> I had never really thought about it like that. It makes a lot of sense, though. So, for that reason you just said about limits of words being the limits of somebody's world, you would say therapists need to be more centered?

Conscious of the fact that we had less than two minutes until the final buzzer was due to sound at 4:30, I try and do Jerry's question some measure of justice.

> I wonder, do conversations require differing levels of centering? For example, when working with a young person of color entangled in the criminal justice system who is afforded very little power, might I have to exercise the power society has given me with the letters and licenses after my name to fight on behalf of the rights of this young person? Might this also require me being 'more centered'? Also, can I be more centered in a way that is not more expert? I worry sometimes that these two ideas might get conflated. And lastly, because I know we're short on time, what if I try and center the conversation? The conversation is a co-creation that couldn't happen without contributions from both of us. In that way I suppose I'm rejecting the notion that either the therapist or the 'client' has to be centered to the exclusion of the other.

I take a deep breath and clasp my hands together at my chest in a gesture of gratitude.

> Okay, I know we're out of time. Can I just thank each of you for your contributions today? It's made the experience more than I could have imagined. Truly. I look forward to seeing all of you again at 9:30 tomorrow morning.

The group returns my gesture of gratitude through affirming nods, smiles, and murmurs of thank you. A line of five people forms at the front of the room. I spend the next 15–20 minutes answering various questions from eager learners. I spend the evening with my hosts at a local restaurant where the conversation, albeit more casually, continues. It is past 10 pm by the time I return to my hotel room. I collapse on the bed with barely enough energy to brush my teeth.

I'm up by 6 am the next morning to go for my customary run. I find that without this, my mind just doesn't have the stamina for a day of teaching. After a quick shower, I head down to the lobby of the hotel where I open my laptop to examine how far we made it in Jane's story. I notice we are perhaps slightly behind schedule. While I initially feel a ping of anxiety in my chest upon realizing this, I quickly remind myself that often the workshops where we 'fall behind' are the ones participants end up saying they find to be of the most value. I've always attributed this to the fact that when participants are really involved, not as much story can be covered.

My hosts drive up outside the hotel lobby at 9 am sharp, and we are quickly en route back to the workshop venue. Returning to the now familiar classroom, the smell of the old building. yesterday's small talk is replaced by conversations about yesterday's work. In fact, the group is so loud that I have to shout just to get everyone's attention and initiate the day's work.

> It's awesome to see all of you again today. I had some time this morning to reflect on yesterday's time together, and my sense is that people are very engaged as evidenced by all of the great questions being asked. Of course, this is just my perception, and I realize that may not be accurate. How are all of you feeling about how this workshop is progressing so far? Should we continue on like we have been or move in a new direction?

The group rather emphatically instructs me to continue down the same path we've been traveling together. I grab a marker and direct our attention to the spirits of practice we had written on the whiteboard yesterday: dignification, wholehearted, flower questions, rebel love, and radical respect.

> As we look at these spirits of practice some 17 hours later, what do you make of them? Can you see how they are showing up in the work, or do you think we may have veered off course?

Helen is quick to respond.

> It's funny because if you would have written all of those on the board at the beginning of yesterday, no offense, but I would have thought you were crazy. I would have been like, what do those have to do with therapy?

The participants nod robustly in agreement. This seemingly unanimous sentiment inspires me to ask a question.

> This is a really interesting point you're making, Helen. What do you think changed? Why do they mean something now when they would have been just weird words or phrases on the board at the start of yesterday?

She takes some time to deliberate, head cocked to the right, before voicing her reply.

> The first thing is the language we used. I think you were right on when you asked us not to use jargon even though I thought that was strange at first. For whatever reason, I remember these better. It's like, oh yeah, rebel love. That's being willing to break rules but for a greater purpose. It's out of this deep care for the person and recognizing how the rules might be holding them down.

My next question flows easily.

> Basically, all of you said yesterday that you were tired of PowerPoints being used to teach as much as they are. Was there anything about the way we arrived at these spirits of practice yesterday that felt like a more preferred way to learn?

Jerry couldn't resist fielding the question.

> You know what's weird? You couldn't have taught us these using PowerPoints yesterday even if you wanted to.

My body leans forward, eager for Jerry to say more.

> How do you mean?

Well, we made up most of those words. How would you know to put them on a PowerPoint ahead of time?

I wonder if the group is stumbling on something at the very heart of the pedagogy.

To be fair, I did introduce the terms 'dignification' and 'radical respect' into the conversation. But all of the other terms came from y'all. And full disclosure, I had no plans to bring up dignification or radical respect. Our conversation pulled them out of me.

Jessica's face flashes a look of astonishment.

So, each time you teach this, it's...different?
If I'm using the same story, there are certainly some elements that will reappear. There's even a decent amount of overlap across stories, but you're right in the sense that I can never be sure what spirits of practice each group will experience in the performance of the story and how they might name them.

The group takes some time to revel in the process we created together during the first day. I join them. After about a 15 second pause, I ask:

Should we dive in and see what today brings us?
We spend a little time inviting our imaginations back into the conversation Jane and I were having and the idea of radical respect. The story touches on Jane's observation that an important consequence of missing the loving and caring sides of one another because of politics can lead to "hate." This leads to the reintroduction of the importance of a third way forward, separate from Republican and Democrat that Jane called "humanness." Then the story begins to take a turn, one that inspired some curiosity in the group.

Do you remember what, I think it was Jerry, said near the end of our time yesterday about how perhaps the radical respect I was trying to practice towards Jane could invite its way outside of just our relationship and how that might be foreshadowing something to come? I couldn't have been more on the same page while in conversation with Jane. Heck, our thinking was so aligned that we may have been in the same sentence!

I begin performing the story again:

> In this moment, part of me wants to bask in the warm glow that experiencing humanness together was bestowing upon us. Another part of me was pleading not to be lulled to sleep by this, insisting that there was more work to be done. In that spirit, I ask, "Do you think it might be important for us to continue to stand up for this third category of humanness in our living out there in the world or should this just be a project for in here?"
>
> After a deep sigh, Jane responds, "I think it will be hard to do it out there. It feels safe to talk about this in here. I know that you won't judge me or think badly of me."

Jessica is quick to make an observation of how this approach is different than some of the formal therapy training she is getting in her graduate program.

> I think it's interesting that you try to move this outside the therapy room. I've been taught that it's just about the relationship between client and therapist and that might move outside the therapy room if it needs to, but there's no way of really doing that intentionally. It's like you're intentionally pushing for this to move outside the therapy room.

I reply with a smile.

> Guilty as charged. Anyone willing to venture a guess as to why I might want to encourage such a move?

Chins sit on fists, brows furrow, and temples are rubbed as the group contemplates an answer. Maya's torso tilts forward ever so slightly.

> It's not just about the individual. It's about the collective.

Feeling that we might be on the verge of something illustrative of the practice, I decide to try and invite Maya a little deeper into her explanation.

> Maya, may I ask, what is your sense of why a collective practice might prove to be of value in this situation?

Maya doesn't appear rushed and measures her words carefully.

> Politics, Republicans and Democrats, exist in groups. That's collective. We adopt these ideas sometimes without even thinking about them. Think about how strong those groups must be for us to do that.

Maya chuckles before taking some time to finish her response.

> Therapy is this little safe room. That's a good thing sometimes, and I think we need that. But that's not where real life happens. Jane needs to explore this out where her real life happens. Otherwise, it's just like a message in a bottle lost in the ocean some place.

The group, as has become its custom whenever Maya speaks, needs some time to digest her ideas. After a protracted pause, I ask:

> Maya, what name might you give this spirit of practice you're talking about?
> I like the word 'collective.'

She speaks in a contemplative tone with her mind still searching for alternatives.

> Communal. How about communal?

A realization provides a jolt of energy to my next question.

> Hey, does anyone else find this even a little bit interesting? Generally speaking, ideas like collective and communal are more compatible with liberal rather than conservative political ideologies, wouldn't you say? For example, if I were to ask her to be more communal, do you think that she might have sniffed that out as something more liberal even if didn't intend that?

I wonder if I can even answer the question that I just posed.

> Can I find a way of asking questions that invite us to consider a communal spirit in a way that doesn't get tangled up in party politics? Perhaps we can evaluate my attempts at doing so? To be honest, I haven't ever thought about this until right now.
>
> I write the word "communal" on the whiteboard despite the challenge it is presenting me in trying to understand my conversation with Jane. We soon encounter a question to evaluate.
>
> *What could our country out there learn from our relationship right now?*

I wonder what the attendees might make of my question given where our conversation has been going. I feel trepidation having never explored this previously.

> What do you make of this attempt to invite a communal spirit in a way that might disentangle itself from party politics?

Helen is quick to advance a response.

> You used the word 'country.' I think that's important because, at least to me, implies everyone could learn from this. Like you didn't say, 'what could a specific political party learn?'

Bella advances the idea further.

> You're also saying that the country could learn from this humanness that you and Jane are creating together. So, the whole country could learn from something being created by a Hillary supporter and a Trump supporter.

A sense of relief comes over me as I realize my question was at least somewhat effective in doing the work I challenged myself to do just a few minutes earlier. After observing Jane's positive response to my questions, the group expresses interest in a direction I choose to explore.

> *I add in a playful but honest tone, "I mean, it's safe to say that our differences still exist, right? We didn't get rid of those?"*
>
> *Returning the playful smile, she replies, "Oh, no! They definitely still exist."*
>
> *I continue, knowing there might be some risk in moving this direction, "Have we discovered that part of this work involves learning to sit alongside differences rather than to eradicate them?"*
>
> *What do you mean?*
>
> *I continue without losing momentum, "Have you noticed that often when two people of different political persuasions get together, they spend all their time together trying to convince the other one to come over to their side?"*
>
> *"Yeah, ain't that the truth," she says vociferously.*

Helen gives voice to what the group seems to be wrestling with.

> You had this kind of positive direction going with her, like you got on the same page together or something. I think it was really interesting that you brought the differences that you have with her back up.

I take a moment to admire the profoundness with which the group is engaging the nuances of the conversation with Jane.

> This is a really sharp observation, Helen. My thought here is that if a counter story is too clean, it makes me a little nervous. Look, the differences that Jane and I share are complex, don't you think? There's no reason a counter story, a story that runs counter to the master narrative of Republicans and Democrats hating each other, can't maintain some complexity. What would be the consequences of not allowing us to acknowledge and maintain our differences? Can we still forge humanness even without agreeing on everything? Do we risk creating a fairytale if we don't incorporate our differences rather than a rich story that could exist in the cold political world we are both required to exist in once we leave the warm confines of my office?

There is a certain heaviness to the group that feels different than what we've experienced together so far. A look of consternation overtakes Jessica's face. Sensing that we have formed a little bit of a bond as a result of our interactions from yesterday, I take a risk.

> Jessica, I notice that you might be having a bit of a reaction to what we've just talked about. I know I could be wrong here, but do you mind if I ask what's running through your mind? If you'd rather not share, just tell me.

Jessica lets out a sigh.

> What you've said makes a lot of sense to me. It's just that it's complicated, like you said. I guess I'm just used to therapy being straight forward. Like there's a set of directions to basically follow.

She pauses with a look of deep concentration still on her face.

> Jessica, is it possible that you are thinking that maybe narrative therapy doesn't have those directions or the manual to follow?

Her face expresses a little more life.

> Yeah, exactly!

> This might sound like a weird question, but do you find the lack of a narrative manual to be a good thing or a not so good thing?

Jessica gives a quick shake of her head, a grimace affixed to her lips.

> I don't know. I mean...it's both. I like the manual because it makes me feel like I know where to go. But...it's like it tries to force everyone into the same box and that obviously doesn't work.

I suspect a pivotal moment in our time together has presented itself. I take a few seconds to measure my words.

> What if instead of writing a manual, we let our narrative spirits of practice guide us in this moment?

Jessica cocks her head slightly, still a bit mystified.

> I just don't know how that would look.

It feels as though my teaching abilities are being stretched about as far as they can go.

> Is it alright if I try and offer a little guidance here?
> I walk up to the whiteboard and write, "Appreciation of complexity." I turn to face the group with a mysterious energy brewing. I am encouraged by memories of when I took risks like this that paid big dividends in prior workshops.
> Alright, I was thinking we might do this a little bit later in the day, but I'm going to throw caution to the winds. Would it be alright if I gave all of you a challenge? I want to give you two spirits we've created together, 'radical respect,' and the one I just wrote on the board, 'appreciation of complexity.' I would like to invite all of you to let those spirits kick around in your consciousness for a little bit and then see what questions they lead you towards.

A collection of skeptical eyes stare back at me. I remain undeterred. I read back a section of the story we had been discussing:

> *I add in a playful but honest tone, "I mean, it's safe to say that our differences still exist, right? We didn't get rid of those?"*
> *Returning the playful smile, she replies, "Oh, no! They definitely still exist."*

237

My excitement only continues to build.

> Okay, what I'd like to do is invite you to ask a question to Jane, guided by radical respect and appreciation of complexity. Don't overthink it. Just see where those two spirits take you. Why don't we each write our questions down. Don't worry, I won't mandate that anyone share their questions. I will, however, provide us opportunities to share should people want to. Does that sound okay?

While still somewhat suspicious, the group slowly begins to step into the activity. I sit down, remove my tablet, and engage in the same task. After three or four minutes, I inquire whether the group has had enough time. After they indicate they have, I stand back up eager to see what they have come up with.

> Would anyone care to share a question that merging radical respect and appreciation of complexity led them to?

A familiar silence overtakes the room. It's one I had heard a number of times over the years when I invite learners to begin practicing. It's taught me to wait out the discomfiture. After about 30 seconds, a few giggles break through. Finally, it becomes so excruciating that Jerry breaks the silence. His narrative therapy experience seems to bring some comfort to the group.

Jerry clears his throat.

> Okay, here goes. If we keep listening to these differences, could they take us to places neither of us have ever been?

I am grateful for Jerry's willingness to break the ice.

> Yes! What a cool question. Jerry, can you help us locate radical respect and appreciation for complexity in your question?

My question appears to challenge him as Jerry is slower in responding than I was becoming accustomed to.

> Hmm... that's a tougher question than I might have guessed it would be. I guess there is respect and complexity in listening to differences.

Would you say that differences usually encourage listening or do they encourage something else?

He offers a reply without delay.

Differences usually make people more standoffish.

Jerry accentuates his words by folding his arms, sitting back in his chair, and scowling.

I open my arms as a gesture to extend my question to all of the attendees.

Would it be fair to say then that allowing difference to inspire listening to one another and leading to new places is radically respectful and complex?

Flickering eyes tell me the ideas are likely resonating.

Is there anyone else who has a question they might like to share?

Helen momentarily occupies the spotlight.

How have we found a way for difference and humanness to exist at the same time? It is possible difference and humanness aren't as different as we thought?

I feel energized by the proficiency of the questions.

Wow! There's a lot to consider here, Helen. I love how you moved to obliterate a potential dichotomy there of difference and humanness. Like if we maintain difference, perhaps there's this assumption that we minimize humanness. Isn't this an example of what we were calling a flower question yesterday? Also, I love your play on words in saying that maybe differences aren't that different. David Epston is a master at wordplay in his questions, and I think it can open up so much possibility. Thank you for this!

Bella's raises her hand in a deliberate fashion. I nod my head for her to proceed. She takes a deep breath.

If differences continued to be our teacher, what wisdom would it teach us?

239

A quiet and excited chatter makes its way through the room with the participants beginning to marvel at their capacity to ask questions. I take a moment to share in the experience.

> You know, you just started composing questions you might ask Jane and, I mean this sincerely, you might already be asking questions better than the ones I asked. Should we see what direction I decided to take?

I take a moment to allow myself to reenter the story before I begin reading the question that I actually asked Jane.

> *"Do you suppose that the fact we don't agree in some ways politically could actually add something to our relationship and the work we're doing that we couldn't access if we had the same political beliefs?"* I ask. *"Might it actually in a weird way be helping us locate a humanness in one another we might not find if our beliefs were similar?"*

The group appears eager to discuss with multiple hands already in the air. I'm left with the unenviable task of choosing a speaker. The group defers to Jessica, perhaps having a sense that she hadn't had a chance to speak in a while.

> The question you asked here really hit me hard...in a good way. I know I'm being taught in grad school that maybe there are some clients we should just refer out to someone else and sometimes that's because of the differences in beliefs we might have about the world or politics or whatever. It seems like you are saying that it could be a good thing that you're different.

I nod in agreement as Jessica is speaking. Maya then picks up where Jessica left off.

> I agree. Maybe it could be a good thing that the two of you are different. Are you saying that the work you are doing with Jane couldn't be done if you had the same beliefs?

I pause and rub my goatee in thought before answering Maya's question.

> At the very least, I'm speculating that it might be true that the different beliefs we hold might allow us to go to a place we couldn't if we held the same

> beliefs. I'm certainly willing for that idea to be vetoed by Jane. This might sound weird, but I don't listen to much political talk radio hosted by pundits I agree with. When I listen, it's almost always ideas that are different from mine. Most of my friends get angry after 30 seconds of listening, and they wonder why I'm not equally outraged. I tell them that I'm just listening with a curiosity to try and understand how people end up formulating the ideas they do. To be honest, I very rarely change the opinion I hold. But I do gain a better understanding of why certain ideas might make more sense to certain people. This also makes me ask questions of the ideas I hold dear. I notice that this understanding helps take me places I may not have gone without it. I guess I might be putting this idea to the test a little bit with Jane.

Helen is nearly falling off the end of her chair with impatience to contribute.

> And then you bring up the idea of humanness, like the fact you are different and going down this road together might help you locate a different kind of humanness. That idea is so interesting to me. What kind of humanness do you think it is?

I notice my enthusiasm rising to meet Helen's.

> That's such a great question, Helen! And to be honest, at this point in the conversation with Jane I'm wondering the very same thing. I would be lying if I told you that I knew exactly what this kind of humanness was at this moment. I was more operating on a hunch I guess you could say. My hope was just that it would end up being a different kind of humanness than the kind either of us was accustomed to.

I take a quick peek at the clock and see that it is already 11:15.

> Yikes! I'm sorry that we've gone on so long without a break. Why don't we take one now? Will 15 minutes be okay? Maybe we can meet back here around 11:30?

As the participants scatter in all directions, I head out the back door and go for a walk around the block that is now starting to feel familiar.

> There's no way we're going to get through the whole story,

I utter under my breath to no one in particular. I begin racking my brain how to plan to deal with this challenging reality and notice the tempo of my steps increasing. I shake off the urge to try and devise a strict gameplan and instead make a pact with myself to let the remaining time take us where it needs to go.

After taking my customary seat on the table at the front of the room, I make an effort to regain the attention of the group. I summon us back into the story. A question arises that Jane and I agreed to live with between meetings:

> *What if between now and the next time we meet we keep an eye out for the way humanness is finding us in the world, most especially with people that we might otherwise not see eye-to-eye with?*

As I read on in the story, the group is fascinated by how this question follows me between meetings with Jane. In fact, it's on my trail with such persistence that it finds its way into a local coffee shop with me and causes such a distraction that I almost failed to place an order. Jerry astutely observes:

> It's almost like that question followed you as much as it followed her.

His observation makes me pause.

> This really has me thinking, Jerry. You know, I've often observed that good questions will get under the skin of people and travel with them, sometimes for the rest of their lives. Why would this be any different for therapists? I think a lot of the questions that get raised in the conversations I have with people do follow me with every bit as much zeal as they do the person I'm speaking with.
>
> As the third meeting I have with Jane in the story begins, the group is keen to consider the fact that she brings up the anxiety that had brought her to see me months earlier since it is not something she had discussed much at all. She describes the anxiety as "melting away."
>
> "What's your sense of why it's disappeared, Jane? Do you think it has anything to do with what we've been talking about in our conversations or perhaps something different altogether?" I lean forward eagerly awaiting her response.

Helen catches something in my question.

> Can you speak to why you brought up the idea of the change being from something else?
>
> I would be happy to. Before I do, can I ask what it is about this that interests you, Helen?

I smile before adding,

> My guess is you didn't bring this up randomly.

Helen returns the smile.

> No, it's just that I wonder why you didn't talk about it just within the context of the work you are doing with her.

I provide a quick thank you nod to Helen for humoring my request.

> You know, I think I might have done exactly what you're describing a few years back, but people have taught me that change happens for all sorts of reasons. Sometimes it's mysterious, random, unpredictable. I'm content that I won't always know why a certain change happened and that such a change won't always be because of something I said or did in my mighty therapist's chair.

I broaden my shoulders in a feeble attempt to look majestic.

As we jump back into the story, Jane attempts to explain why she believes the anxiety might have started to subside despite the fact we hadn't been discussing it. She comes to the realization that fear of judgment was linked to the anxiety that routinely visited her. Excitedly, Jane then shares an account of a lengthy conversation she had with a woman, named Deborah, who was a Hillary supporter and who lives down the street. This turned into a dinner with their respective husbands.

The attendees were all leaning forward, appearing to be firmly in the grip of the story.

> "Do you mind if I ask if the topic of Trump or Hillary came up?" I ask this question with a little bit of hesitation but also a sense that I owe it to our work to broach it.

243

> *No, it never did. It's not like I was avoiding it or something. It's just that there were more interesting things to talk about.*
>
> *The wall of judgment and politics would try and convince you that these differences must define the conversation, but somehow humanness helped you find a different direction?*
>
> *Yeah, I guess that's right. It turns out that we actually have a lot in common. We both have adult sons. We both like to garden. We both have the same taste in music. And my husband and her husband really get along, too. I was almost a little embarrassed that it took me this long to get to know her.*

The group seems generally satisfied with how my conversation with Jane is progressing. I suspect they might see a 'happily ever after' just around the corner. I, however, know the curveball that awaits. It's the kind of curveball that can make any baseball player flail away as though they had never swung a bat before. I feel a nervous yet still somewhat excited energy brewing in my gut.

After accepting some compliments regarding my questions, I read on in the story.

> *Jane, do you think this newly forming friendship you are creating with Deborah could withstand the realization that the two of you voted for different people?*
>
> *"Are you saying I should tell her?" I feel a little extra sting in Jane's words.*
>
> *I remain silent with hopes that Jane takes some time to further evaluate this prospect. Jane continues, "I mean, what if she gets angry or won't talk to me anymore?"*
>
> *This certainly comes with risk, doesn't it?*

It's as if the participants can begin to feel the winds shifting. A few people in the room wince with discomfort at where the conversation is headed. I feel it important to give voice to this.

> I wonder, is bearing witness to this conversation helping along some uneasiness?

No one else in the group verbally acknowledges the unease, but sometimes silence says things words can't. I push forward.

> Would it be alright if I let you know that I'm not particularly proud of my contribution to the next portion of the story I'm going to read? If I had to do it over again, I certainly would have done it differently.

The group looks as engaged as I have seen them in the two days we've spent together. I wonder to myself what it is about tension that can be an asset to learning. I read on, sharing my next query to Jane regarding her relationship with her new Hillary supporting friend, Deborah:

> Can this humanness the two of you have created together get you through this challenge much the same way it helped us get through?
>
> "Maybe, but she's not a therapist. What if it goes totally differently? What if she isn't as nice to me as you were?" Jane bounces her right leg nervously, the muscles in her face strain.
>
> Do you have some sense that because I'm a therapist I might have gone easy on you with regard to trying to reconcile our politics?
>
> Jane pauses. The pressure in the room is now bearing down on my head, much the way it feels during an ascent to 30,000 feet in an airplane.
>
> "It's not like I think you were lying or something," Jane asserts, "but it is your job to be nice to me, right?"
>
> "Is that my job?" I reply quickly. I feel like a shortstop that just made a throw and now wishes he could have it back moments after it leaves his fingertips.
>
> "I guess not." Jane's tone is sullen.

I pause to check in with the group. Knowing that they might not want to offend me, I feel it important that I take more of the lead in facilitating this particular conversation.

> Has anyone else had a question that just sort of flew out of their mouths that they wish they could have back?

The participants nod in solidarity.

> If I had to do this over again, I wish I would have inquired with genuine curiosity about what Jane meant by 'nice.'

I take a moment to try and cobble together a question on the spot.

> For example, something like, 'Jane, I've come to learn that "nice" can mean a lot of different things to different people, when you use the word nice here, can you help me understand what it means?' Instead, I just kind of operated, rather hastily I might add, on what I presumed she meant by 'nice.' I think

245

> that can be a rather dangerous way to proceed and led to what could have sounded like a curt question.

I pause to take stock of the room and invite the group back into the conversation. Jessica looks eager to give her perspective.

> I really appreciate what you just did. You know, I feel like I make mistakes all the time, but I'm just a beginning therapist. I've never really had an experienced therapist show me mistakes that they make. It seems like they just sit on the other side of the mirror and tell me all the mistakes I make.

A certain onerousness forces its way into the room. Jessica's voice cracks as she tries unsuccessfully to continue speaking. As she begins crying, Maya, sitting directly adjacent to her, comforts her with a grandmotherly hug. It feels as though Maya's arms are so long that they extend to comfort all of us. My own remembrances of feeling like a failure as a grad student in much the same way Jessica described come flooding back.

> Can I share a little secret with you, Jessica? I can't think of a single conversation I have with someone where I don't spot things I could do differently. If I ever arrive at a place where I look at a conversation that I've had with someone and see it as perfect, do you think that might be the moment that I become dangerous?

Jessica cocks her head slightly to the left.

> What do you mean?

My response is quiet and intentional.

> When I lose the ability to critique my work, the possibility that it is operating in a way I don't necessarily want it to, increases. The longer that is allowed to fester, the more damage it has the potential to do. And if my work is above scrutiny, how can I with a straight face invite anyone else to take a deeper look at their work alongside me?

I pause to gather my thoughts a little more firmly.

> I wonder if there are a set of ideas operating here that define a mistake as being bad, or as being made by a person of poor character? As a nod to my friend Jane, what if we defined a mistake as simply a consequence of being human?

Jessica raises her head slowly and says through tears with a wry smile:

> I just wish you could get my supervisor onboard with this.

The group responds with a hearty collective laugh.

> This isn't easy, is it? You know, this has me thinking of the work of Vikki Reynolds.[2] She talks about something called the supervision of solidarity. It's really powerful work. I would encourage each of you to check it out. I suppose the conversation we're having now is my small, initial attempt at practicing what she refers to as 'relational ethics.' I hope it represents me using the power I have been granted in a way that welcomes a more humane, egalitarian, and reciprocal form of critique.

I take some time to test the temperature of the room and see if we might move back into the content.

> Would it be okay with all of you if we talked a little bit more about the particulars of the thicket that I led Jane and me into?

The group gives me their assent.

> Jane brings up the idea that maybe my job as a therapist is to be nice to her. I quickly, and perhaps unthoughtfully, ask if that is my job. Now, to be fair, I'm not upset with the idea itself. I think I should have a conversation with her about whether or not my job is to be nice. However, what burns me as I read it aloud to you even now, is that I said it so tersely. I take pride in trying to be thoughtful about the language I use and how I use it. I don't think I was very thoughtful here. It leaves me feeling a bit off-kilter in the time before our next meeting. In fact, I'm wondering if perhaps I might have derailed our work. When she starts the next meeting by saying, 'Thanks,' I was positively confused!

I feel a strong desire to continue reading the story that deflates quickly when I look at the clock and notice that it is lunchtime.

> Well, perhaps this is as good a time as any to stop and get some sustenance in our bodies. Should we meet back here at 1:30?

As the participants head for the exits, I sit quietly in the front of the room. I feel a strong sense of gratitude and exhilaration that is simultaneously tempered with a touch of sadness knowing that I only have three hours let with this group. It always seems no matter how much time I have with a group of learners, I am always craving more. I try to silently reassure myself. If there is no melancholy at the end, then it probably wasn't worth anyone's time. Not feeling particularly hungry, I opt to gnaw on a protein bar while I go for a walk.

I arrive back in the classroom with about 15 minutes to spare. The room is largely empty with just a couple of people pecking away on their devices, headphones on, adrift in the digital world. I resist the urge to pull out my phone. Just be a person for a second, I whisper to myself. A couple minutes later, Jessica returns from lunch with a couple of her fellow participants. She approaches to initiate a conversation. The decibel level in the room gradually increases as more people trickle back in.

> You remember what you asked me at the beginning of the workshop yesterday about seeing if things start to make more sense?

Jessica's back straightens and she speaks with conviction.

> Well, I do. I was just telling my friends at lunch that I feel like I understand narrative therapy better than I ever have before. When I read the textbook about it in my class, I was...just really confused. I liked some of the ideas, but it was like it was way over my head.

I smile knowingly at Jessica.

> Would you believe that I felt the very same way when I was first introduced to narrative ideas in 2004? Don't get me wrong, I loved the ideas. But they were way over my head, too! May I ask what it is that has narrative therapy resonating with you today?

Jessica measures her words carefully.

> My wife and I are building a new house together, and we recently got the blueprints. Those mean nothing to me. I just can't imagine what it will actually look like. My wife? Her brain works in a way that she knows just what it will look like. She's already planning where she will put furniture. To me, it's just a bunch of blue lines on paper. That's what narrative therapy was to me before these two days. But now, this workshop has actually built the house and I can see it and walk around in it. It has brought it to life.

I find myself hanging on each word as it exits Jessica's mouth. I am rendered momentarily speechless.

> Uh... just wow. I'm not sure I have the right words to tell you how much your words mean, Jessica. I can't imagine a better outcome for a workshop like this than what you just described. Some day when we write a book about contemporary narrative therapy, can I just let you write the little blurb on the back that tries to convince people to buy it?

We both share a warm laugh together.

> Now, hopefully I don't screw it all up in the next three hours!

Time has totally gotten away from me. We're five minutes past due to get going. The room is as loud as I've heard it in the last two days. I wave my arms in vain and momentarily wish I was an aircraft marshal with the handheld illuminated beacons to grab the group's attention. After a couple more failed attempts, I finally corral the eager learners.

> I want to make sure we maximize our chances of getting to the end of the story we've been working on. Is it alright if we get going again? I believe we left off in the story with me being quite worried about the way in which I asked Jane if my job was to 'be nice' to her in therapy. This worry traveled with me between meetings, and I was quite shocked when she began our next meeting by saying thank you. Does that sound about right? And remember, all of this related back to whether or not Jane might talk to her new friend Deborah about their political differences.

The group confirms my account, and I begin reading the story again. They appear eager to discuss the following exchange in more detail:

> *You pushed me to try and talk to Deborah about our politics, and you know, it was the right move.*
>
> *I'm fixated on her use of the word push fearing that it might confirm one of my worst fears. "Yeah, you know, Jane, I've been thinking a lot the past couple of weeks. I've wondered if perhaps I pushed too hard? In fact, I wish I would have done more inviting than pushing."*
>
> *Oh, I don't mean to say that I felt pushed like against my will or something like that. What I mean is that you helped me push through a hurdle I might not have pushed through by myself. It's almost like the way a personal trainer would help someone run a little harder than they might want to, you know?*

Without hesitation, Helen initiates the conversation.

> *I think that's the radical respect we were talking about again. She said it was the right move, and you were still concerned that she used the word 'pushed.' You could have just been satisfied that she said it was the right move, but you weren't.*

I lean back slightly and run my finger against the stubble on my cheek, pondering Helen's words.

> *Even just hearing you say the word 'pushed' now, Helen, makes me squirm a little bit. It just sounds so forceful. I don't want to make a habit of pushing people. As it turns out, Jane was using the word a little differently, but I think I owed it to her to check this out.*

As I continue reading, ever cognizant of the ticking clock, we arrive at another passage the group is enthusiastic to discuss.

> *What about this conversation you had with Deborah made the relationship feel more real?*
>
> *Jane's body leans into the conversation a little bit more. "It boils down to can you like me, who I actually am? I've always felt that I had to be this specific person for everyone else. Basically, like the perfect person for them."*
>
> *Did it feel as though you had to be many different perfect people depending on who you were interacting with?*

> Jane's energy is now indisputable. "Yes! I've been trying to be so many different people. After this conversation it's like I could just be one version of me."
> And would you say that this is the version of you that you like most?

Multiple hands make their way skyward after my last question. Jerry makes a confession.

> Sometimes I read ahead of where you're reading on the screen. I'm not trying to be rude or anything.

I give a face of faux outrage that draws scattered laughter.

> You're not the first person to admit this to me, Jerry. I don't mean to be presumptuous, but I've come to know you a little bit over the past couple days and I have a hunch you are sharing this right now for a reason.

Jerry grins while continuing.

> It's just that in the next paragraph, Jane begins crying. As I was reading this a certain word came into my mind, and it's a word that has come into my mind before with narrative therapy 'Liberation.' I feel like that last question is the moment she might be starting to feel liberated from perfectionism.
> The small vibration of a buzz in the room can be felt tingling our feet after Jerry's observation. I write the word "Liberation" on our board.
> Thanks for this, Jerry. You've invited me to think about a lot of different things simultaneously. I'll start by saying that I wonder if sometimes it's not a single question that helps move people, but maybe a sequence of questions? To be honest, it was my hope that I might be able to help disentangle Jane from perfectionism. If you walk back three or four questions, though, each one is building toward where the last one took us. For example, imagine if I would have just asked the question, 'Would you say this is the best version of yourself?' directly after Jane told me the relationship with Deborah felt more real. I would argue that this question might not have had the same impact. I want to extend what I hope would be a fun challenge to each of you. What would it be like to look at your questions not as isolated entities, but rather, as interconnected? The essence of the current question can never be fully understood without looking at the questions, and responses, that led up to that question.

Not wanting to get lost in this idea, which was surely one we could spend all of our remaining time exploring, I endeavored to pivot back to another gem Jerry handed us.

> I'm happy to talk more about sequencing of questions with any of you later on, but I want to make sure we try and do justice to the notion of 'liberation' that Jerry brought up. Does that resonate with anyone else?

Maya lifts her left arm at a near ninety-degree angle, index finger extended. The group eagerly awaits her contribution.

> Liberation is at the heart of narrative practice, at least the way I understand it. There are ideas that can dominate people. It was this liberation element, that I really didn't see in any other therapy in the same way, that drew me to narrative therapy.

I feel almost a duty to continue building on Maya's words.

> You know, what you and Jerry are both saying, Maya, is also something that attracted me to narrative ideas. I often work with people who are being imprisoned, sometimes literally, by master narratives about who people should be. Contemporary narrative therapy is not afraid to directly confront issues like racism, sexism, and so on. In the case of Jane, what are the master narratives you think we might be confronting?

The group takes some time to rack their brains. Bella is the first to advance a response.

> I think for people, women especially, there is an expectation to be perfect. Where do you think that idea comes from?

The participants remain pensive. Helen adds with a smile:

> Probably from men, and probably heterosexual men, since they have usually had more power.

The rest of the group seems to be a bit stumped about how to build off of Helen's words. I feel it might prove helpful for me to take the lead.

> I think you're onto something here, Helen. Might I add something else that I think is in alignment with your idea? I wonder if, and I'm sorry for the jargon here, but the ideas of neoliberal capitalism are peddling this notion of perfectionism, which most certainly encompasses patriarchy as you indicated. For example, Ronald Purser wrote this really interesting book entitled *McMindfulness*. I really love how he talks about neoliberalism. He defines it as a type of cultural and economic dominance where decisions are left up to the marketplace. This then positions everyone as in competition with everyone else, effectively running their own, what he calls, 'business of Me.' I wonder if this positions us as always in comparison to others, and thereby, not good enough. In this system, there can literally be only one person on top. This leaves the rest of us feeling like we must always get better. Might this infect people with a kind of perfectionism that has us running on a treadmill and no matter how fast we run, we never seem to get there?

Jessica looks distressed upon hearing my words.

> Yeah, so it's like we are never good enough. We can never really accept ourselves.
>
> Acceptance might be great for the act of being a person, but I'm not sure it's so good for keeping an economic engine churning.

I flash an ironic smile.

> To me, one of the big challenges of what we're calling contemporary narrative therapy is not just to understand the ideas we are talking about right now, which are quite philosophical in nature, but to be able to turn those ideas into inquiries. We also owe it to learners like each of you that we speak in a language that can be understood by most anyone. I mean, I can wax philosophical about neoliberalism all day, but I'm not sure that does the people who consult me a whole heck of a lot of good. Nor does it position narrative therapy as a way of working that most people feel like they can actually practice in a forum like the one we've shared together the past couple of days.

I call for our last break. The pressure of time is bearing down on my chest in a way I hadn't felt all weekend. I am pondering the fact that there is so much more I want to explore with this group. How does one do this work justice in two days? I take one last jaunt around the block. I arrive back in the classroom, urgency biting at my heels.

> My hope is we can put a bow on the story here in our last hour together. You know, while I was going for a little walk, I was thinking about how much more we could do together if we had another couple of days. Of course, if we had four days together, I would probably be wishing we had six. Maybe that's just kind of how these things go, huh?
>
> The group meets my words with an abundance of warm smiles. It reinforces the feeling that perhaps what we have done the past two days has been of some value. I settle into the home stretch of the story in which Jane and I revisit the anxiety that originally brought her to see me. Jane notices that when she can "just be me" the anxiety seemingly evaporates. The work begins to come full circle.
>
> *Do you think we could have discovered this if you and I had the same political beliefs or we didn't have the conversation about politics that we had a few weeks back?*
>
> "I really don't think so," she says firmly. "I thought I was going to come here to see you for anxiety and you were going to give me some techniques or something to fix it. I didn't think that who we are as people would even matter. I mean, I had never done anything like this. But this is so much deeper. To know that you actually like me despite that we voted for different people helped me learn something I didn't even know I needed to learn."

The group now almost effortlessly interacts with the story without me having to deliver many cues or prompts. Helen shakes her head a bit before speaking.

> What sticks out to me here is her saying that she learned something she didn't even know she needed to learn. That's powerful.

I respond quickly with a question for the participants.

> How the heck do you think we got to this powerful place together?!

Jessica continues in the rhythm of the conversation.

> I think it's because you were willing to take a risk together. It goes back to... what did we call it?

Jerry interjects:

> Rebel love.
> Yeah, rebel love,

Jessica replies with an energy shining in her eyes.

> I was all freaked out about this when we talked about it yesterday, but now I see how that risk paid off. It makes me wonder what would have happened if you didn't take this risk.

I can hardly contain my excitement.

> Jessica, remember how you said you had no idea how to implement our spirits of practice and all that? Can I share something with you? The thought you just had of what might have happened if we didn't take that risk, that's exactly what I was thinking when I was speaking to Jane! Now, I'm not saying that you must think what I'm thinking or that it's the only way to think, but don't you think it's interesting that we are both having the same thought in this moment?

Pride subtly lifts Jessica's shoulders and chin just a little higher than they had been yesterday.

> Jessica, I'm operating on a big gut feeling here, and I don't want to put you in a bad spot. Please feel free to decline my invitation and I won't be in the least bit offended. I'm just wondering, might you feel comfortable offering a question you would like to ask Jane about letting the spirit of rebel love lead the way?

Jessica's cheeks puff out as air whistles quickly through her pursed lips. She takes some time to study the last exchange Jane and I had that was still on the screen, but as of yet unable to see the next question. Her fellow students patiently wait in suspense.

> Okay, here goes,

Jessica takes a deep breath.

> Do you...

she stumbles over her words. The group urges her to continue, assuming a stance of solidarity.

> You got this, girl,

Maya says with conviction.

Jessica nods her head as if she was letting Maya's words penetrate her being. She recollects herself and delivers her question for Jane:

> Do you think the things we need to learn most are those things we didn't know we ever needed?

The group erupts with oohs, ahhs, and claps. I find myself clapping as well. Jessica looks pleased, but given the red hue of her cheeks, also a touch embarrassed by all the hoopla.

Jessica than serendipitously adds a follow-up question:

> What is over and behind the hills of the things we never knew we needed to know?

The group collectively gasps with intuitive appreciation.

> You know, I come to this conclusion time and time again when I'm teaching like this and someone utters a question like the one Jessica just did. It never fails that the group responds like we are right now with a sense of excitement and awe. And can I tell you something, Jessica? I would pay good money for those questions in that moment. Those are as good as any question I could have asked. I really mean that. In fact, I'm quite certain those are better than the question I actually asked. Do you think those questions came more from your head or from you heart?

Jessica's head quickly rocks backwards a few inches as though it was in some way jolted by my question.

> Wow. No one has ever asked me that before... I would have to say my heart. It's not like I really thought about it at all. You said to let that spirit of rebel love guide it. Once you said that, it's like the question just came to me.
>
> Hold on just a moment,

I reply as I scroll down on my computer to reveal the question that I actually asked so that I can read it aloud.

> *Jane, do you think these ideas we've discovered in here are better than ideas we might have found in a book or on Google?*

I take a moment to get reacquainted with my question before speaking.

> You know, my question is fine. I think it gets the job done. But Jessica, just listening to your question and given that it came from your heart in the way you described, I think your question has more 'duende' than mine. Have you all heard that word before, 'duende?'

A collection of puzzled eyes stare back at me.

> Okay, don't worry. I hadn't heard the term either before my friend and colleague marcela polanco introduced me to it. To be honest, I'm still trying to understand it at the level I would like to.

I momentarily pull out my tablet to look up a quote that I think might come to our aid.

> Give me just a second,

I say as I try and swipe to the digital promised land.

> Oh, yeah. Here it is. It's a quote from Federico García Lorca.[3] 'The duende, then, is a power, not a work. It is a struggle, not a thought. I have heard an old maestro of the guitar say, 'The duende is not in the throat; the duende climbs up inside you, from the soles of the feet.' My question talks about books and google searches. It might be clever in some way, but it doesn't make the people in the room react the way your question did, Jessica. This is why I say I think your question has more duende. Now, not every question can have duende, but I might suggest that duende is at the heart of what contemporary narrative therapy is trying to accomplish.
>
> Duende momentarily sweeps me away from worrying about time or outcome but time is quick to knock on the door and remind me of its presence. We begin reading the final couple pages of the story and stumble upon a

257

conversation about "magic." Jane tells me about her love for the book *The Minpins* and a particular quote that goes as follows: "Those who don't believe in magic will never find it." That serves as inspiration for the following exchange:

This is a major guess on my part, so I know I very well could be wrong here, Jane. But do you think we might have located some kind of most unlikely magic in here?

Jane takes some time to metabolize my question more fully. "Well, I figured you'd done this sort of thing with other people like me before. Maybe not exactly the same, but you know, like pretty close."

Can I tell you a dirty little secret, Jane? I've never done this kind of work we've done together with anyone before. And, to be honest, I'm quite certain I couldn't have pulled it off without you as my fellow trailblazer.

I see Bella's head cock just slightly, and I wonder if she might have something to say. I look her direction, and she accepts my invitation to speak.

So, you mean you *really* never did this kind of thing with someone before?

I let out a little chuckle.

No, I honestly hadn't. Long before I knew this might become a chapter in a book, I began writing it up mostly just to try and explain it to myself. I got to the end of it and Jane reported that it made a big difference in her life, but I really had no idea exactly why. I would say in general each meeting I have with someone is different, but there can certainly be common elements. This, however, was like nothing I had ever done before.

Helen flashes me a look of kind impatience.

Okay, well did you learn why it worked?
 That's a very fair question. I'm not trying to dodge your question here, but can I share with you what Jane said? I think she might be able to say it better than I can.

I take a quick glance at the clock and see we have less than ten minutes left and read aloud one of our final exchanges in the story.

If you were to summarize what it is about this work we've done as a whole that will stick with you and that you might not be able to get out of your head or your heart, what might that summary include?

> *If someone that is supposed to hate me can invest this much in me, maybe I'm not such a bad person. Maybe I'm okay. Maybe we are okay?*

I notice tears welling up in the eyes of a couple of the participants. I'm swept back into this final chapter of my work with Jane as though I'm experiencing it anew. I can simultaneously taste the bittersweetness of my two-day workshop with this group coming to an end. All of that is enough to stop any words from immediately needing to be spoken.

After a collective respite, I use the remaining precious minutes to finish the story. The group claps. We cross the finish-line with nary a minute to spare.

> I'm happy to stick around if people have additional questions, but I want to be respectful of your time and let you get out on the roads as I know traffic will likely get bad quickly. May I just make one last invitation? If any of what we've done here in the last two days follows you into your work and you have time, would you be so kind as to write me and let me know about it? And if was not helpful at all, I'd certainly be up for that feedback, too. I'd just like to know how it has impacted you – good, bad, or indifferent.

A line of people forms to say thank you, ask lingering questions, and exchange contact information. Some 30 minutes later, the room has finally cleared out. I sit down in the chair adjacent to the whiteboard where our spirits of narrative practice came to life. I admire what we were able to accomplish together, so much so that I feel sadness at the prospect of erasing them. I read each spirit one last time:

Dignification
Whole-hearted
Flower Questions
Rebel Love
Radical Respect
Communal
Appreciation of Complexity
Liberation

Not a bad list at all for two days, I say to myself. I remove my phone, hit the camera icon, and snap a quick picture of the board. I walk toward the exit and turn off the lights knowing that this workshop will travel with me in ways that I probably can't yet understand.

Over the course of the next couple of months, I received emails from a few of the participants updating me on how the workshop was influencing their work. Each one was exhilarating in its own way. However, the words of Jessica are what still stand out. She wrote:

Dear Travis,
I can't thank you enough for the workshop last month. I want you to know that I feel like it changed my life. Never has narrative therapy looked so crystal clear to me. It's weird because I feel like even though the workshop was only two days, it's given me more than my graduate school training has in two years.

So, you said to write and let you know if anything from the workshop was coming into our therapy sessions. Well, I want you to know that I ask flower questions like nobody's business! I feel like I've become at least decent at asking them. I was working with a couple and they talked about how they argue all the time. I think they just immediately expected me to judge it as bad, but that's when the spirit of the flower question bloomed for me. I asked, what do you mean when you say arguing? Is there arguing that is helpful for the relationship and other kinds of arguing that are not? Just like we were talking about at the workshop, it opened up all kinds of petals that we could take a look at.

Another spirit that I've been trying to carry with me is radical respect. I really like that one. For me that's the taken the form of, how can I show respect to this person in a way that maybe they have never experienced it? The example I can think of, and I don't know if it's a good one, is I am working with a ten-year-old boy. Everyone at home and at school was using the word 'hyper' to describe him. I realized between meetings that I was doing that, too. That's when I thought of how you had worried that you had pushed Jane instead of inviting her. You were talking about stories traveling with you, well, let me tell you, that one sure traveled with me. The next session, I apologized for using the word 'hyper' with him and asked him if he would like to use a different word. At first, he looked at me like I was crazy. Then he came up with the idea that sometimes his tank is filled with 'excited gas!' This was so much more helpful. To me, this felt like the spirit of radical respect, and I wouldn't have thought I could even do this without seeing how you did something similar with Jane.

Okay, so I'm sure you're busy. I won't take any more of your time. But I just wanted you to know that the way you're teaching is working.

> I've already recommended that my classmates go to one of these workshops. And I want to go to another one, too.
> With ever expanding duende (at least I hope),
>
> Jessica

As I finish reading her words, I have a smile on my face that is soon met with a salty tear that is running down my cheek. I walk out of my office, mind adrift in all the potential adventures that might lie ahead for contemporary narrative therapy.

Notes

1 From Ludwig Wittgenstein (Author), C. K. Ogden (Translator), Bertrand Russell (Introduction), *Tractatus Logico-Philosophicus* 471st ed. Edition, London: Dover Press.
2 Reynolds (2014) Centering ethics in therapeutic supervision: Fostering cultures of critique and structuring safety. *The International Journal of Narrative Therapy and Community Work*. No. 1, 1–13.
3 "Teoría y juego del duende" ("Theory and Play of the Duende"); Maurer (1998) pp. 48–62.

CHAPTER 9

CONCLUSION

A Literary Means to Pedagogical Ends

Tom Carlson

In November 2019, I arrived a day after Travis at David and Ann's home in Auckland where we were to spend the next ten days collaborating on preparing a draft of this book. Travis and I began each day running for an hour up to the top of nearby Maungawhau (Mt Eden), a 1,000-foot-high ascent and then having breakfast together on our way back. By then, David was eager to get going. David and I would sit beside Travis, who was the designated typist, at the dinner table.

After dinner, we would sit by the fire in the living room and continue, but now it was my turn to take notes on my laptop. To some extent we were preparing for the next day by doing so. One of us would say to the others, "Hey, let's record that for tomorrow," and the delegated spokesperson would dictate his comments and I would record them. Perhaps this made each of us more thoughtful in restating what otherwise would have been considered a very congenial evening's conversation. All of us looked forward to these reviews of the day's writing and even more so to thoughts to be taken up in earnest the next day.

It was an unusually cold November night. We had just finished our last day of writing the book proposal and the first draft of all the chapters for it. The open fire in the living room was already ablaze and warming up the room and the conversation that is about to take place.

"I can't believe that our 10 days together has already come and gone," I said with a bit of melancholy in my voice.

CONCLUSION

"Yes, but can you believe how much work we were able to do by being in the same physical space and putting our collective minds together," David reflected as he sits back in his chair, holding a glass of wine as if a reward for a hard day's work.

"It really is surprising how quickly this book project has come together. Was it April (2019) when we started? And now it is November and we are nearly done," Travis said with a bit of wonder in his voice.

David, never one to let a chance to story our efforts go by, jumped in with a proposal.

> Tom and Travis, maybe it isn't such a surprise given all the preparation that has gone into our pedagogy over the past four years. Perhaps it would be worth our while to think back on how this all started so that we don't lose sight of what it was that kept propelling us forward with this project.
>
> This whole time we have been here together in Auckland, my mind keeps returning to the workshop that we did in Vancouver in 2018 alongside Kay Ingamells and Sasha Pilkington, where we first tried out this pedagogy. Travis and David, do you remember the wonderment and awe that we felt upon experiencing the participants' unusually tender and heartfelt responses to the practice stories?

"How could I forget! It was like nothing I had experienced before. People were coming up with tears in their eyes, holding their hands to their hearts, as if saying 'Thank you,' barely able to speak," Travis said.

> I will never forget, what that one person said. I think it was Ashley who had attended your workshop at the University of Denver, Travis. She came up to us both and fell silent for a moment, as if she was searching for the words that could meet the moving of her heart. And then she said three words that are forever etched in my mind. 'It restored beauty.'

"That's right, Tom," Travis said,

> And do you remember the woman who came up to us and said, 'This presentation, and the stories that you shared, brought the spirits of narrative therapy back to life for me and restored all of my earliest longings and desires for why I became a therapist in the first place.' I have heard similar comments over and over whenever I use this pedagogy.

David couldn't help but join in.

> You know what still has me bewildered, are the outcomes that your students reported from your class, Tom, rating one three-hour class using this pedagogy as being worth eight to 16 weeks of your more classical teaching on narrative therapy. What does that come out to? Three hours of teaching through a single case story is equivalent to 24 to 48 hours of teaching based on theory. I know students can be generous in their evaluations but that's still beyond anything I could ever have hoped for. I know that this was in the context of your graduate class on narrative therapy, Tom, but you and Travis have also tried this pedagogy out in many different teaching formats, including workshops to novices and experienced narrative therapists alike, and the 'results' were similar.

"That's right, David! I remember first telling you both about this and how surprised we were by these early findings. But these 'findings' pale in comparison to their own words about the effects of this pedagogy. As you were talking David, I remembered a particular comment from a student in one of my workshops who emailed me several months later. She said,

> The stories became companions to me in my work with my own clients. In fact, the stories and the people in them seemed to show up when I needed them most. The funny thing is that I didn't have to do anything to conjure them up. I carried them with me in my heart.

David couldn't help but interrupt.

> That's precisely what I had hoped for—that the stories would somehow companion them in their work. I have to give credit to Art Frank for introducing this idea to me. I once heard Art say, in a keynote address several years back, that stories have a unique capacity to serve as 'travel companions' to their readers—as if they become co-inhabitants in the stories—and will spontaneously make an appearance in their own travels with others.

A smile appeared on Travis' face, as if he was in a moment of personal reverie.

> That reminds me of an email I received from a more experienced narrative therapist who participated in a workshop I gave in Denmark. She said that

learning in this way was like 'falling in love all over again' and reminded her of why she was so attracted to narrative therapy in the first place.

Spurred on by the fire, we reminisced for what seemed like hours about these early experiences and how our bewilderment set us on a path to make sense of it all. And then the conversation took a turn. David had been unusually quiet for a while. His eyes gazed into the fire as if the fire was conversing with him. Travis and I decided to join him in the silent conversation of his mind.

Then David broke the silence.

"Tom and Travis, I can't tell you how pleased I am to see this come to fruition. I have to admit that I felt some apprehension at the ways in which narrative therapy seemed to become more and more de-spirited. The more I think about it, the more I have come to the conclusion that it wasn't so much the maps of narrative therapy, or even the one-page version that it has been reduced to, but rather it is the required obedience to the maps as the right way of doing narrative therapy. Let me find the quote that Michael and I wrote in the introduction to Epston and White (1992) on experience, contradiction, narrative, and imagination, which was our source for the idea of the 'spirits of practice' and perhaps this very project itself. Here it is..."

> With regard to ideas and practices, we do not believe that we are in any one place at a particular point in time, and rarely in particular places for very long. In making this observation, we are not suggesting that developments in our work are sharply discontinuous- they are not. Nor are we suggesting that our values and our commitments are varying- they are not ... However, we are drawing attention to the fact that one of the aspects associated with this work that is of central importance to us is the spirit of adventure. We aim to preserve this spirit, and know that if we accomplish this our work will continue to evolve in ways that are enriching to our lives, and to the lives of those persons who seek our help.
>
> What will be the direction of this evolution? It could be tempting to make pronouncements about this. But these would be hard to live by. And besides, our sense if that most of the 'discoveries' that have played a significant part in the development of our practices... have been made after the fact (in response to unique outcomes in our work with families), with theoretical considerations assisting us to explore and extend the limits of these practices
>
> (p. 9).

David paused for a moment, looking again into the fire. Sensing that there was much more to come, Travis and I didn't dare to break the silence.

David continued,

> Did I ever tell you about "the googlization of maps" since 2007? Before Google, maps were more like guides or suggested routes. Michael clearly specified this in his introduction to *Maps* and drew upon his experience as a pilot. Let me go to my bookshelf and get it so I can refer to his comments.

David returned with his well-worn copy of Michael's *Maps* in hand. "Here is what Michael had to say about his idea of *Maps* and it comes with a caution:

> The maps that I review in this book are, like any maps, constructions that can be referred to for guidance on our journeys—in this case, our journeys with the people who consult us about the predicaments and problems of their lives. Like other maps, they can be employed to assist us in finding our way to destinations that could not have been specified ahead of the journey, via routes that could not have been predetermined. And, like other maps, the maps that I present in this book contribute to an awareness of the diversity of avenues that are available to preferred destinations… I have formulated these maps over the years principally in response to requests from other to render more transparent the therapeutic process that I have developed. I will emphasize here that the maps in his book are not *the* maps of narrative practice or a 'true' and 'correct' guide to narrative practice, whatever narrative practice is taken to be
>
> (White, 2007, p. 5).

David continued,

> When driving somewhere, people would briefly consult the map to get their bearings but they would make their own determinations about how they wanted to get somewhere. But Google maps changed everything. Michael's untimely death in 2008 meant that he was not there to see his idea of a 'map' be so redefined by what the discipline of cartography calls 'the googlization of the map.' And I think it has very much to do with the de-spiriting of narrative therapy that Michael lamented to me before his

death. With the advent of Google maps, maps are no longer guides to be consulted, maps now require our obedience which goes by the euphemism 'fidelity.' When we use Google maps, we enter the destination, and Google literally tells us when and where to turn and we simply obey. No thinking required. No departures from the pre-designed route. And if you do so, you will be reproached by the bot.

David looked back into the fire and fell quiet again. This time Travis broke the silence.

> This has me thinking about what we are hoping for by teaching through stories. The stories don't tell people what to do. They don't present formulas or steps. They don't tell people, 'Turn left here' or 'Turn right there.' What they do is to place the reader inside the scene, inside the mind and heart of the therapist, and into a feeling relationship with the thoughts, ideas, and practices enacted in the story. The story demands something of them. It asks them to think their own thoughts, to infer for themselves the spirits that guide the work and how the questions that the therapist asks are directly informed by them. I guess you might say that the stories seek to literally bring narrative ideas and practices to life.
>
> David and Travis, I just had a wild thought. You know how we have often referenced E.M. Forster and his notion of flat and round characters? Let me pull up the quote here. Okay, here it is:
>
> Flat characters, in their purest form, are constructed round a single idea or quality. Once they are identified, flat characters never surprise us, never waiver. They do exactly what they are supposed to do, no more and no less. Round characters, by contrast, possess multiple qualities, shadowy ambiguities, and outright contradictions. Most important, they are capable of change
>
> (As quoted in Mattingly, 2010, p. 108).
>
> Okay, so here is the wild idea. What if this idea of flat or round characters were to be applied to narrative therapy itself? Has narrative therapy, through the focus on maps and our obedience to them, developed a flat character? And does this, in turn, have the effect of creating flat therapists? Therapists who do what they are supposed to, who do not waiver from the map, who do not experience surprise and does this mean they end up bereft of their own imaginations."

"That's very apt, Tom," David said excitedly.

> And the whole purpose of the stories is to present a re-inspirited narrative therapy that engages the minds, hearts, and in particular solicits and cultivates the imaginations of therapists; to help them develop into round therapists who are capable of surprise, who can think in novel ways when they have ventured into new territories. I guess it has always been my hope that the stories would encourage readers to find their own way, in their own spirit and by way of their own experience-near vocabularies.

Travis and I nodded in agreement and we settled into our chairs, each of our minds now taking flight into the hazy mix of memory and possibility. Our reveries were only broken when David rose to put a few more logs on the fire: "Maybe tomorrow..." he began.

References

Epston, D., & White, M. (1992). *Experience, contradiction, narrative and imagination.* Adelaide: Dulwich Centre Publications.

Mattingly, C. (2010). *The paradox of hope: Journeys through a clinical borderline.* Berkley, CA: University of California Press.

White, M. (2007). *Maps of narrative practice.* New York: Norton.

INDEX

Note: Page numbers followed by "n" denote endnotes.

abuse: personal experiences of 85; tolerance 73
Adrenalin Forest 72n2
anger 104, 136, 152, 184
anorexia see Wilbur (anorexia, case study)
anti-colonial counseling 222
anxiety 174, 192–194, 196, 198–199, 201, 230, 242–243, 254; and death 26; and fear 106; problem of 20; return of 64–65
Australian and New Zealand Journal of Family Therapy 12
Australian Family Therapy Journal 14
autoethnography: evocative 15, 28, 29, 31–32; narrative practices 23–24, 31; as pedagogy for teaching 23–24; and soul of practice 28–33

Bakhtin, Mikhail 28
Basso, K.: *Wisdom Sits in Places: Landscape and Language Among the Western Apache* 13–14
Bateson, Gregory 28
Behar, R. 15; *Vulnerable Observer: Anthropology That Breaks Your Heart* 15
Bochner, A. 28, 32, 262; *Coming to Narrative: A Personal History of Paradigm Change in the Human Sciences* 28
Bruner, Jerome 12, 15, 28

cancer see Chuan (cancer, case study)
care/caring: institutional 77; and loneliness 124; and loving 232; palliative 117–118; and protection 79, 81
Carlson, T. 34, 35, 151–172, 262–268
The Case of the Nightwatchman (Epston) 14
Chuan (cancer, case study): approaching death 127, 134, 143; challenges of living 133; chemotherapy and its side effects 125, 129; death of 150; and Eastern music 122; effects of steroids 140; expressing sadness 141–143; gifts of young people 137; in hospice inpatient unit 117–118, 146, 148, 149; intimate spiritual experience 123; Kang (son) 117–118, 127, 129–130, 134, 137, 138, 149; kindness 134–137, 144; life experience and Buddha 123; palliative care 117–118; reasons for leaving hospital 147; and Sasha conversations

(*see* Pilkington, S. A.); sense of companionship 124; sense of humor 130–131; Shan (husband) 117–118, 126, 146–149; starvation and poverty, death from 131–132, 135; symptoms 120–121, 145, 148
classrooms 31, 33
Clinton, Hillary 174, 177, 178, 182, 184, 193, 211, 215, 221, 235, 243, 245
Coming to Narrative: A Personal History of Paradigm Change in the Human Sciences (Bochner) 28
contemporary narrative therapy: anti-colonial counseling or cultural democracy 222; anxiety 242–243; appreciation of complexity 237; Bella (counselor) 206, 212, 222–223, 225–226, 235, 239, 252, 258; 'betraying social justice' 223; brand new to 206; communal spirit 234–235; difference and humanness 239–241; dignification 232; 'ethics' or 'values' 209; externalization 207; fear of judgment 243; formal therapy training 233; gesture of gratitude 176, 229–230; Helen (psychologist) 207, 209–210, 213, 216–217, 220, 223–224, 226, 231, 235–236, 239, 241, 243, 250, 252–254, 258; Jane 35, 174, 177–201, 207, 209–211, 214–217, 219–226, 230, 232–236, 238, 240–245, 247, 249–252, 254–260; Jerry (therapist) 206–208, 211–212, 214–215, 217–220, 226–229, 231–232, 238–239, 242, 251–252, 255; Jessica (participant) 207–210, 212, 214, 216, 218, 221, 232–233, 236–237, 240, 246–249, 253–257, 260–261; long history with 206; Maya (participant) 209, 211, 213–214, 220, 224, 233–234, 240, 246, 252, 256; 'radical respect' 224–226, 232, 237–239; Republicans and Democrats 236; risk 218–219; rules in therapy 217–219; self-disclosure 212; 'spirits' of practice 207–210, 221, 230, 237; success of workshop 213; use of language 213, 228; using Power-Points 231; value of Heidi's observation 215
counseling 41, 63, 97, 111, 117, 170, 193, 206, 222; anti-colonial 222; multicultural 222

counter-mapping, process of 22
couples therapy (Megan and Dan, case study): acceptance of relationship 164–165; anger and resentment 152; appreciation of experience of partners 170–171; awareness of special relationship 166; 'demoralizing' and 'draining' 158; emotions and love 154–155, 162; force of conviction 159; hope and conviction 156; living with distance and quiet resentment 156; moment of honored silence 160–161; physical and verbal responses 151; proud of relationship 169; sense of self-worth 157; shared craziness 167–168; shared memory 159; sign of liveliness 154; surprise meeting 172; verification of love 163
critical cartography 22, 266
cultural democracy 222

Dahl, Roald 199
depression 76, 113, 120–121, 216
distress 47, 61–62, 78, 114, 141, 148, 253
Duvall, Jim 12

eating disorders 34, 41
Ellis, C. 28, 32
Epston, D. 3–16, 17, 21, 28–29, 31–32, 34, 73–82, 229, 239, 262–268; *The Case of the Nightwatchman* 14; Mother Appreciation Parties 73–82; *Playful Approaches to Serious Problems: Narrative Therapy with Children and Their Families* 3
Erickson, Milton H. 11
evocative autoethnography 15, 28, 29, 31–32
exemplary tale-book 13

Fabiola 34; "the ability to trust" 88–91; achievements 115; activated kind of trust 91; anxiety and fear 106; conversation summaries 101–104; "juvenile stunts" 109; kind of hatred 96; 'leadership role' 97; "little girl" 111; mistreatment by "exes" 114–115; moments of fear and doubt 112–113; *pièce de résistance* 106; "quietness" or "soft-boundaried-ness" 97; refusal of rights 95–96; remembrance of

Index

counterhistory of voice 97–98; resolved voice 93–94; Restraining Order 96, 105; struggle and honesty 88–89; trip to New York 106–108; voice 99–101; "Why me?" 85–87

fear: absence of 68; and doubt 112; getting rid of 70; of heights 60; of judgment 243; worst 196, 250

Forster, E.M. 15, 267

Freeman, J.: *Playful Approaches to Serious Problems: Narrative Therapy with Children and Their Families* 3

García Lorca, Federico 257

Google maps 266–267

Grasseni, C. 23; "skilled vision" 23

habit of "freestyling" 17

hatred 110, 152, 164, 167, 186–187, 200, 232, 259

Heath, T. 17–18, 35, 173–201, 203, 205–268

Huerta-Lopez, Ana 29

humanness 232; counsel 193; and difference 239; third category of 187, 233

Ingamells, K. 34, 263; Wilbur (case study) (*see* Wilbur (anorexia, case study))

Ingold, T. 23, 31

Jane (contemporary narrative therapy, case study): admission of voting for Trump 35; "breakthroughs" 178; and Deborah, friendship 194–196, 198, 245; human category 184, 187; humanness 193, 232; political category 179, 181, 185, 191, 195; 2016 Presidential election 211; radical respect 224–225; revelation of 214; social justice 201; theory 192; therapeutic vitality 200

Journal of Systemic Therapies 12

Julie (Mother Appreciation Parties, case study): Beth (friend) 79; Brandon (son) 73; "emergency responding" 75; husband's overseas trips 73–74; as "just plain dumb" 76; post-party meeting 81–82; private and secret meeting 79–80; relieve of distress 78; "surprise mother appreciation party" 78–81; "temper tantrum party approach" 76–77; tolerance of abuse 73

"knowing your limits" concept 5–10

Lacoste, Y. 20

literacy, practices of 14

Lobovits, D.: *Playful Approaches to Serious Problems: Narrative Therapy with Children and Their Families* 3

love 137–138

Mair, M. 28

Manen, M. van 15, 16

Mannering, Simon (New Zealand rugby player) 72n1

manualized approaches 11, 19–20

maps: critical cartography 22; Google maps 266–267; "googlization" of 19–20, 266; manualized approaches 19; narrative 19–20, 265–266; non-manualized approaches 19; notion of 19–20; prevalence of 24

Maps of Narrative Practice (White) 19, 22, 266

Mattingly, C. 14

Matulino, Ben (New Zealand rugby player) 72n1

Maybe We Are Okay: Psychotherapy in the Time of Trump 32

McMindfulness (Purser) 253

mother appreciation parties

multicultural counseling 222

My Voice Will Go with You: The Teaching Tales of Milton H. Erickson (Rosen) 11

narrative maps 19–20, 265–266

narrative therapy: contemporary (*see* contemporary narrative therapy); couples therapy session (*see* couples therapy (Megan and Dan, case study)); practice stories 12; practitioners, training students as 20–21; re-inspirited 268; searching for story in 25–27; "spirit of adventure" in 17

non-manualized approaches 19

oral cultures used stories 13

271

Paljakka, S. 34, 84–115
palliative care 117–118
Pilkington, S. A. 34, 117–150, 263
Playful Approaches to Serious Problems: Narrative Therapy with Children and Their Families (Freeman, Epston and Lobovits) 3
"poetizing form of writing" 16
polanco, marcela 29, 257
practice stories: genre of exposition of practice 12; "in the moment" storytelling approach 1; narrative therapy literature 12; as a puzzle 11
The Process of Questioning 12
professionalized storytelling 26
psychotherapy 28, 33, 177, 201, 213
Purser, Ronald E. 253; *McMindfulness* 253

Rosen, S. 11; *My Voice Will Go with You: The Teaching Tales of Milton H. Erickson* 11
Ryle, G. 23; "knowing that" and "knowing how," distinction between 23

Sacks, Oliver 28
self-disclosure 175, 211–212
social justice 183, 201, 221–223, 222
"the spirits of practice" 23, 29, 208–209, 221, 230–232, 237, 255, 265
Staring at the Sun (Yalom) 25–26
storytelling 1, 13, 26, 28, 31, 211
supervision of solidarity 247

"temper tantrum party approach" 76
therapeutic conversation 24, 26, 28–29, 203
therapy rooms 24, 32, 74, 233; children adjoining 74

therapy sessions 43–72, 91, 99, 101, 151, 161–162, 166, 169, 217, 260
Thompson, Nick 14
transcripts 24, 25, 27, 28, 207, 217
Trump, Donald 35, 174, 177, 178, 181–185, 191, 193, 194, 197, 201, 203, 215, 221–223, 225, 235, 243

Vulnerable Observer: Anthropology That Breaks Your Heart (Behar) 15

White, M. 12, 14, 17, 19, 20, 32, 265; *Maps of Narrative Practice* 19, 22, 266
"Why me?" (Fabiola): poetic version 86–87; standing ovation 85
Wilbur (anorexia, case study): assessment 42; childhood worries 41; Doug (father) 42, 44–45, 47–48, 50–52, 54–57, 59–60, 62–72; hair pulling 48; intentions to rescue people 46; legendary imagination 69; Liz (mother) 41–48, 50–51, 54, 61–62, 64–65, 71–72; and music 47, 72; playing instruments 72; responsiveness 50; a rugby jersey 46–49; session five 66–72; session four 62–65; session one 43–50; session three 57–61; session two 51–56; as a 'Sheep Worrier' 51–56; soccer and cricket 47, 72
Wisdom Sits in Places: Landscape and Language Among the Western Apache (Basso) 13–14
Wittgenstein, L. 16, 229
workshops 11, 29–33, 35, 203, 205–206, 213, 217, 222, 228, 230, 237, 248–249, 259–261, 263–264

Yalom, I. 25, 26; depictions of therapy 26; *Staring at the Sun* 25–26

Made in the USA
Monee, IL
04 March 2025

13399043R00157